≈ ≈ ≈

The Anti-Inflammation Diet and Recipe Book

About the Author

Dr. Jessica K. Black graduated cum laude from Cardinal Stritch University in Milwaukee, Wisconsin, in 1998. She received her medical degree from the National College of Naturopathic Medicine in Portland, Oregon, in 2002. Dr. Black now lives in Portland, Oregon, and enjoys running both locations of A Family Healing Center with her husband, Dr. Jason Black. They have one beautiful daughter, Sadie Rae. Apart from her work as a naturopathic physician, Dr. Black enjoys hiking, biking, skiing, and eating good food in the company of friends and family.

DEDICATION

❧ ❧ ❧

This book is dedicated to my beautiful
daughter, Sadie Rae Black.

Sadie,
Thank you for teaching me patience, the value
of playing, and how to love unconditionally.

Ordering

Trade bookstores in the U.S. and Canada please contact:

Publishers Group West
1700 Fourth Street, Berkeley CA 94710
Phone: (800) 788-3123   Fax: (800) 351-5073

Hunter House books are available at bulk discounts for textbook course adoptions; to qualifying community, health-care, and government organizations; and for special promotions and fund-raising. For details please contact:

Special Sales Department
Hunter House Inc., PO Box 2914, Alameda CA 94501-0914
Phone: (510) 865-5282   Fax: (510) 865-4295
E-mail: ordering@hunterhouse.com

Individuals can order our books from most bookstores, by calling (800) 266-5592, or from our website at **www.hunterhouse.com**

The Anti-Inflammation Diet and Recipe Book

Protect Yourself and Your Family
from Heart Disease, Arthritis,
Diabetes, Allergies — and More

Jessica K. Black, N.D.

Hunter House Inc., Publishers
PO Box 2914
Alameda CA 94501-0914

Library of Congress Cataloging-in-Publication Data
Black, Jessica.
        The anti-inflammation diet and recipe book : protect yourself and your family from heart disease, arthritis, diabetes, allergies-and more / Jessica Black. — 1st ed.
                p. cm.
        Includes bibliographical references and index.
        ISBN-13: 978-0-89793-485-5 (pbk.)
        ISBN-10: 0-89793-485-7 (pbk.)
        ISBN-13: 978-0-89793-486-2 (spiral)
        ISBN-10: 0-89793-486-5 (spiral)
        1. Inflammation—Diet therapy—Recipes. I. Title.
RB131.B58 2006
641.5'6318—dc22   2006020190

Project Credits
Cover Design: Brian Dittmar Graphic Design
Book Production: Hunter House, Blair Cavagrotti
Developmental and Copy Editor: Kelley Blewster
Proofreader: Herman Leung
Indexers: Robert and Cynthia Swanson
Acquisitions Editor: Jeanne Brondino
Editorial & Production Intern: Blair Cavagrotti
Editor: Alexandra Mummery
Customer Service Manager: Christina Sverdrup
Order Fulfillment: Washul Lakdhon
Administrator: Theresa Nelson
Computer Support: Peter Eichelberger
Publisher: Kiran S. Rana

Printed and Bound by Sheridan Books, Ann Arbor, Michigan
Manufactured in the United States of America

11 10 9 8 7   First Edition   10 11 12 13 14

Contents

*detailed recipe listings for each section are given on these pages

Foreword

One's individual choice of foods for themselves and their families has a great deal of effect on day-to-day health, as well as on prevention of chronic health problems. This is well recognized and documented in today's scientific world.

Many years ago, in my work with patients, it became evident to me that most people ate on a daily basis foods that were not good for them. When they made dietary changes and no longer ate food allergens or foods to which they were sensitive, they invariably began to feel better. Through years of experience and with the help of nutritional science, I was able to devise diets that helped most patients. From this evolved the anti-inflammatory diet recommendations.

When people need to change their diets, the most common question is always, "Well, then, what do I eat?" Fifteen years ago it was almost impossible to find acceptable substitutes for many of the common food allergens or foods that have been shown to cause chronic inflammation. Recipe books contained many of the foods that I was recommending people avoid, so they were forced to just try on their own to make substitutions and then hope the recipe "turned out to be edible."

Dr. Black took it upon herself to come up with delicious recipes that require no (or few) substitutions. Just follow the recipe and, voilà, a masterpiece. The tried and proven dishes you are about to discover will delight any discriminating palate. Jessica's work at preparing and testing the recipes on friends and relatives has resulted in a must-have cookbook. As a bonus, her recipes include nutritional information about the content of fats/oils, protein, and carbohydrates, as well as other vital nutrients.

More than just a cookbook, this text is a guide to help you learn how to cook healthfully and to appreciate the tastes of healthy eating. This book will simplify your work in the kitchen. Jessica has recipes for everything from breakfast items to appetizers, side dishes, salads, soups, main courses, and desserts. All these tasty recipes meet the criteria of low-allergen, anti-inflammatory food choices. Changing one's diet, preparing healthy meals, and enjoying nutritious foods were never so easy.

Over time you will want to try all the recipes offered in this book. You will have your favorites, but as your palate expands so will your level of health and wellness. Jessica shows that healthy eating need not be time consuming. Quick and efficient—yet nutritionally sound—meal preparation can now be a reality for everyone. You can prepare these meals after a long workday and be extremely satisfied.

Dr. Black has done an incredible job of creating a book that will enhance your eating pleasure. Give yourself and your family the greatest pleasure you can at mealtime by eating healthy foods and following the recipes outlined in this book.

Happy eating.

— Dick Thom, D.D.S., N.D.
Portland, Oregon

Preface

I truly loved preparing the food for this cookbook. Because I love cooking and love keeping myself and my family healthy, writing this book became a necessity so others could get the same satisfaction from cooking that I do. My husband and I are strong proponents of living healthy lifestyles, and we strive to impart our philosophy to as many people as we can. We figure if we can educate others, they in turn can educate the next group of people, and through the wonders of small talk we can create a collectively healthier population.

Have you ever noticed that when you are in a good mood and feeling fine, the people around you seem to catch on to that energy and good things just begin to happen? And, similarly, have you noticed that when you are not feeling well or are feeling a little angry or grouchy, people around you can sense that energy and in turn begin to feel or act negatively as well? If we allow ourselves to live day in and day out not feeling well, we and the people around us suffer, including our family members and children. Conversely, if we begin to take charge of our health through proper diet, exercise, and positive thought, our well-being and the well-being of all the people around us seem to improve.

Paying attention to our health and using natural medicine is a great new trend in our society. It is easy to get excited about health as you begin this diet, because everyone who follows it sees some positive change. The diet was developed with the idea of reducing overall inflammation in order for the body to work more efficiently. (Why should we focus on reducing inflammation? For an answer to that question, see Chapter 2.) As naturopathic physicians, I and many of my colleagues recommend this particular diet to every patient. I have seen arthritis patients reduce their pain by 50 percent (or more), people with allergies become allergy free, and sufferers of chronic diseases receive hope—all from the health improvements these patients notice upon beginning this diet. In addition to improving health in general, the anti-inflammation diet allows the treatments people follow to work better because overall metabolism and bodily function have improved.

What prompted this recipe book was the need of all my patients to determine what to eat once I had suggested a new diet for them. Transitions are tough, but they seem to be even more difficult when people don't know how to change or what to eat to facilitate the change. I kept one food-allergy cookbook in my office that I found myself lending to my patients, with frustration that I didn't have twenty more copies to go around. At each visit I offered my patients more and more dietary suggestions. Finally I decided to write them all down in an easy-to-use and inspiring cookbook.

Part One of the book lays the foundation by explaining the concepts behind holistic health and naturopathic medicine, the importance of reducing systemic inflammation, and the basics about the anti-inflammation diet. Part Two contains the recipes. Each recipe offers a relevant tidbit of health information. Most recipes also offer ingredient substitutions to help you as you experiment in your kitchen.

Congratulations on your choice to begin a new, healthier way of eating. At times, making the transition may be difficult, but remember that you are affecting more than just yourself; by following the anti-inflammation diet you are contributing to a healthier world. Let this book be a blessing to all who use it, let it inspire new ideas, and let it guide you on the path toward vibrant health.

Acknowledgments

First I must offer my gratitude to my husband, Jason Black, N.D. Without his input, I might have included some recipes in this book that may not have been to anyone's liking. I give all my love to you, Jason, for always inspiring me to try something new, for truly teaching me to *love* food, and for sharing my passion for preparing the most elegantly beautiful life-giving foods. Thank you for continually challenging me to become a better healer and better person.

I want to thank many of my colleagues for creatively showing up at potlucks with dishes I had never dreamed of. It is so hard to name them all, but when I think of unique dishes, I seem to think of Matt Fisel, N.D., Chelsea Hunton, MSOM, Erika Siegel, N.D., L.Ac., Heidi Lescanec, N.D., Kristen Lum, N.D., and many others. Words cannot describe what an incredible experience medical school was because I was surrounded by so many talented, intelligent, spiritually gifted, and zealous individuals.

I want to thank Debra Passman, N.D., for showing me how to love and crave sushi outings, and Sarah Vlach, M.D., and Mark Holbrook for the entertaining sushi-rolling nights essential to keeping my love for sushi alive. I especially want to thank Wendy Abraham, N.D., for always being the best friend and colleague anyone could ever have or want. Special thanks also go to my good friend Stephanie Findley, who has diligently accepted the anti-inflammatory diet into her household and has tested many of the recipes in this book for me.

Special thanks close to my heart go to my family for being supportive as I trudged through an unconventional school to receive an unconventional degree to learn an unconventional way to cook and live. I appreciate my family for embracing and respecting my profession as much as I have grown to love and respect all of my naturopathic mentors and colleagues.

Last, but not least, I thank Dickson Thom, D.D.S., N.D., for teaching me the true way of healing and for willingly sharing his incredible knowledge of nature cure. Thank you for introducing me to the anti-inflammatory diet and to the profound results it can have on health and vitality.

Important Note

The material in this book is intended to provide a review of information regarding an anti-inflammation diet. Every effort has been made to provide accurate and dependable information. The contents of this book have been compiled through professional research and in consultation with medical and health professionals. However, health-care professionals have differing opinions, and advances in medical and scientific research are made very quickly, so some of the information may become outdated.

Therefore, the publisher, author, and editors, as well as the professionals quoted in the book, cannot be held responsible for any error, omission, or dated material. The author and publisher assume no responsibility for any outcome of applying the information in this book in a program of self-care or under the care of a licensed practitioner. If you have questions concerning your nutrition or diet, or about the application of the information described in this book, consult a qualified health-care professional.

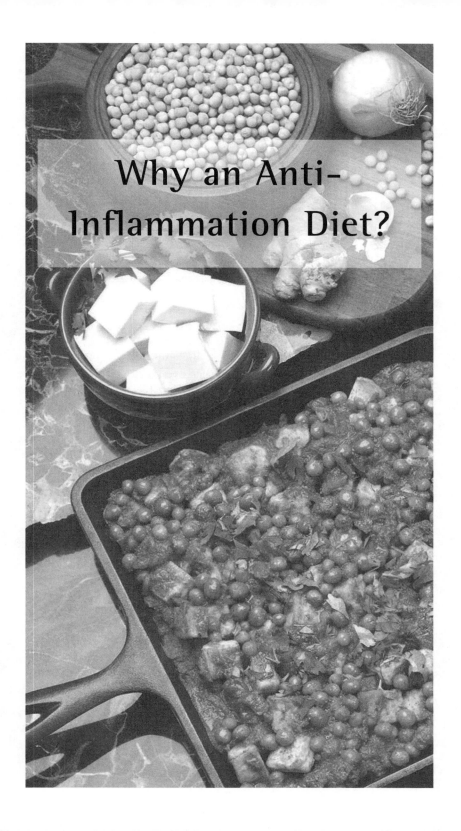

Why an Anti-Inflammation Diet?

❧ ❧ ❧

Modern
Health Paradigms

The art of healing comes from nature, not from the physician.
Therefore, the physician must start from nature, with an open mind.

— *Paracelsus*

The current American lifestyle causes a large amount of concern among people who care about health. There has been a dramatic increase in noncommunicable diseases within the last decade, and that number is still rising. According to the Centers for Disease Control and Prevention (CDC), seven out of every ten deaths are attributed to chronic diseases such as cancer, diabetes, and cardiovascular disease (e.g., heart attack and stroke), all of which have a direct nutritional connection.

Right now at least two paradigms of healing exist in our society. One paradigm, which centers around diagnosing and treating disease, takes a mechanistic approach to illness in which the patient's symptoms are combated with pharmaceuticals and/or surgery. This approach assumes that if the patient's symptoms improve via painkillers, antibiotics, steroids, or other suppressive treatments, then the patient is cured.

A second paradigm, the one embraced by naturopathic medicine, looks at a person as a whole and acts to stimulate his or her healing, even before disease is apparent. This paradigm, of which prevention is the cornerstone, strives to maintain homeostasis within the body, allowing it to function optimally and thereby promoting improved health. Disease symptoms function as messengers to tell us what is going on in the body and can direct the practitioner to treat certain systems to bring about better health. Disease merely indicates the existence of a "disease" in the body—that is, an imbalance. When symptoms appear, they are only the tip of the proverbial iceberg that for some time has been developing beneath the surface. This paradigm approaches symptoms as indicators of something going on deeper in the body; rather than merely suppressing the symptom, it strives to find and remove its true cause.

The Role of Primary Care

In recent years the federal government has stated that primary care is the ideal setting in which to provide nutritional education to the public. However, according to an article published in *Family Practice* in 2000, many primary-care doctors are reluctant to educate patients due to their disbelief that dietary intervention can be a worthwhile modality, despite the fact that numerous studies exist showing positive dietary influences on health outcomes. For example, a randomized, controlled trial published in July 2003 by the *Journal of the American Medical Association* found that adding soy protein, viscous fiber, and nuts can be as effective for lowering cholesterol as adding a prescription statin medication to a low–saturated fat diet.

Another article published in the *New England Journal of Medicine* in 2002 stated that diet and exercise may be more effective than pharmacologic therapy at defending against cardiovascular diseases in patients with impaired glucose tolerance. After three years of making diet and lifestyle changes, patients decreased their risk of developing diabetes by 58 percent. In contrast, participants who were only taking metformin, a common pharmaceutical prescription for diabetics, reduced their diabetes risk by only 31 percent. This is a significant difference. In addition, participants following the lifestyle changes had a significant reduction in C-reactive protein (CRP), which is an indirect marker of subclinical inflammation. (Subclinical inflammation is inflammation that can't be detected through the usual diagnostic procedures. The role of inflammation in health is the topic of the next chapter.) Metformin participants affected their CRP levels significantly less than lifestyle-change participants. These findings are huge breakthroughs for diabetic patients—if they get the information.

Naturopathic physicians are recognized primary-care physicians. In states where they are licensed to do so, they provide lifestyle and diet-modification education in a primary-care setting and actively teach prevention strategies. Naturopathic physicians offer dietary intervention because they believe in it completely. Many naturopathic physicians have seen their patients experience significant health improvements through diet, lifestyle change, and various other naturopathic modalities.

As a naturopathic physician, it is my duty and goal to educate my patients about how to change their health by changing their lifestyles. I help to put the power of healing into their own hands. The body has the innate wisdom to heal itself; sometimes it just needs a reminder to stimulate its own healing. We like to say that everyone has her or his own inner doctor. A few wise choices in lifestyle habits can change one's quality of life immensely. We just need to take better care of our vessels, and they can do amazing things on their own.

What Is Naturopathic Medicine?

A licensed naturopathic physician (N.D.) attends a four-year, graduate-level naturopathic medical school and is educated in all of the same basic sciences as a medical doctor (M.D.), with the difference that he or she also studies holistic and nontoxic approaches to healing, with a strong emphasis on disease prevention and optimizing wellness. A naturopathic physician is board-certified by his or her state and is expected to uphold the highest standards of primary medical care. Currently, fourteen states, the District of Columbia, and the U.S. territories of Puerto Rico and the U.S. Virgin Islands license naturopathic physicians to practice primary care. When searching for a naturopathic physician in states that do not have licensing procedures, it is important to find out about his or her credentials. Make sure you are being treated by a properly trained physician who has attended a four-year, accredited, postgraduate naturopathic medical school. There are currently four such schools in the United States and one in Canada. For more information on finding a naturopathic physician in your area, you can contact the American Association of Naturopathic Physicians or Canadian Association of Naturopathic Doctors (see Online Resources, in the back of the book).

Naturopathic medicine is successful at treating various acute and chronic diseases. It excels in treating chronic illness when allopathic medicine has nothing left to offer. In acute conditions, it often supports the body's own natural healing mechanism. Some common conditions treated by naturopathic medicine include, but are not limited to, allergies, asthma, anxiety, depression, fatigue, digestive complaints, skin complaints, autoimmune diseases, thyroid problems, menstrual irregularities (including menopause symptoms), acute colds and flus, chronic infections, and cancer.

Services offered at a naturopathic clinic vary depending on the physician but may include acute care; women's medicine; I.V. therapy including chelation (an intravenous injection of ethylene-diamine-tetra-acetic acid, EDTA, an amino acid that eliminates heavy metals and other elements from the body and that has been used to improve metabolic function and blood flow through blocked arteries); wellness; pediatrics; physical medicine and spinal manipulation; nutritional counseling; homeopathy; drainage (a specific form of cellular-level detoxification); and botanical medicine, with a focus on chronic disease and cancer support.

Naturopathic medicine is no secret. As naturopathic physicians we seek to help the body begin to restore health and maintain homeostasis. We pay attention to all aspects of the patient's body, mind, and spirit to ensure balance in all of these areas. Often, simple dietary recommendations or a few lifestyle changes begin to turn the body around. At other times we need to help the body direct itself in a certain way by supporting specific systems with vitamins, minerals, botanicals, homeopathy, or other natural medicines.

The underlying principles of naturopathy that help so many individuals achieve optimal health are listed below:

- First, do no harm.
- Identify and treat the cause.
- Impart the healing power of nature.
- The doctor is teacher.
- Always treat the whole person.
- Emphasize prevention.

If everyone were to live by these principles, rates of illness and premature death would decrease significantly.

How Disease Begins

When the body is able to stay in balance and avoid being subjected to any "dis-ease," then it stays healthy. When something happens to disrupt the body's equilibrium, or homeostasis, it becomes more susceptible to disease. Many physiological and psychological factors affect the balance within the body and therefore affect the body's susceptibility to disease.

According to Henry Lindlahr, M.D., from the book *Philosophy of Natural Therapeutics,* "One of the primary causes of disease is an abnormal composition of blood and lymph." Blood and lymph are responsible for transporting nutrients to the tissues, essentially feeding their functions, and for carrying away wastes, toxins, and metabolic byproducts to be excreted from the body via the liver and kidneys. The composition of these fluids is solely dependent upon what type of lifestyle practices we follow and what type of nutrients we bring into the body via diet to fuel the vital body processes.

It follows, then, that diseases are often the result of nutrient deficiency, resulting in the delivery by the blood and lymph of less than adequate amounts of nutrients to fuel cell metabolism. This in turn is the result of an inadequate, unbalanced, or polluted diet. According to Lindlahr, if the diet consists of an excess of low-quality proteins, carbohydrates, and fats, tissues will inevitably be clogged with "morbid matter." This "morbid matter," or toxin accumulation, can interfere with vital cellular functions, thereby becoming pathogenic to many systems in the body. The buildup of toxins in turn supports cellular degeneration, moving the system toward disease, rather than supporting the cellular regeneration needed for healing.

Depending on the constitution of the individual and on his or her ability to eliminate accumulated wastes, diseases can manifest in many different forms. One individual may experience skin rashes, allergies, and asthma, whereas another, who is less efficient at eliminating wastes, may store waste products in the form of cysts, growths, and eventually cancer. Only when the body is properly balanced can it function optimally, including adequately removing wastes.

The Flaw in Germ Theory

Louis Pasteur is responsible for bringing our awareness to the fact that certain microorganisms cause certain diseases. This is the Pasteurian germ theory of disease. For example, Pasteur noticed that diphtheria bacillus is found in diphtheria patients, and thus he concluded that diphtheria bacillus causes diphtheria. Yet diphtheria bacillus can be found in a healthy throat as well. The same can be said about many diseases, including strep throat, staphylococcus infections, pneumonia, whooping cough, and so on. In each of these instances, the same microorganisms can be found in a healthy individual who has been exposed to the germ yet does not contract the disease. The Pasteurian theory that bacteria cause disease simply cannot pass the test of modern research.

Two mentors of mine, Dr. Dickson Thom, a naturopathic physician practicing in Portland, Oregon, and Dr. Gerard Gueniot, a holistic medical doctor from France, have always taught that disease is only able to affect a body that is susceptible. When a body is no longer in homeostasis for any reason—for example, improper diet, poor lifestyle habits, genetic family history, chronic emotional stress, environmental toxin overload, or sedentary lifestyle—it becomes weaker, rendering it less able to defend itself against certain microorganisms and other disease states. We call this general state of bodily reactivity and health one's "terrain." Based on the strength of one's terrain, disease can be either avoided or inevitable. According to Dr. Rene Dubos, renowned microbiologist at the Rockefeller Institute for Medical Research, "Viruses and bacteria are not the cause of the disease; there is something else. Most human beings carry throughout life a variety of microbial agents potentially pathogenic for them; only when something happens which upsets the equilibrium between host and parasite does infection develop into disease."

This means it is not the bacterium or virus that affects us; it is the upset equilibrium that weakens our resistance, thereby allowing disease to occur. Regardless of what we call this equilibrium (or homeostasis or terrain or susceptibility), what we are speaking of is the body's ability to remain disease free.

The Health of Our Children Equals the Health of Our Future

If we have a strong belief in maintaining a healthy terrain, it follows that we want to promote health in our children. As children grow bigger and stronger, the insides of their bodies are also developing in important ways that we are unable to see. Children's nervous system, brain, and immune system develop throughout childhood. To promote optimal health and development, it is important to protect children's terrains through proper diet and lifestyle. If we focus on minimizing pesticide residues, hormones, and antibiotic residues in foods; including nutritive foods as part of a balanced diet; eliminating food allergies; and eliminating sugars, white flour, and other immune-suppressive foods, children will be much healthier in the long run. If we promote a healthy lifestyle from the start, many children will remain disease free. I believe it is my responsibility to my child to keep her healthy in order to prevent future chronic disease. It is also important to offer children a loving, supportive atmosphere in which to grow and develop, because as you will learn in chapters to come, emotions play an important role in health and disease.

There is one more thing to note about children's development. When a child is faced with a bacterial or viral insult and gets a cold, flu, or fever, it is a positive reaction. It allows us to see that the child's body is able to react against foreign antigens. It is important for children to get sick and to mount fevers a few times per year. As this happens, the immune system is "practicing" and developing. In our medical practice we often observe that after a child has gone through an illness, he or she will do something new. He or she may say a new word, take his or her first step, learn a new skill, act with a little more conviction about things, or build more self-confidence. This is a truly amazing aspect of childhood development; children develop as their immune response develops. If we damp down the immune response with Tylenol, antibiotics, or any other suppressive treatment, we are telling

My daughter, Sadie. Our children can inspire us to make lifestyle choices that promote health, so that we can pass those good habits along to them.

Photo credit: Jessica Black, N.D.

the body not to react and thus not to practice developing its immune response. If we suppress children's reactions enough times, the body will stop reacting.

The immune system has many components, and if all components are not exercised and developed, the system can become out of balance. The child whose immune response has been suppressed too often may stop having minor infection reactions such as colds and flus, which are the body's way of fighting against bacteria, viruses, and any other foreign material it is exposed to. Decreasing the proper reaction of the immune system in children allows them to be exposed to many foreign invaders that are never fended off. If these invaders are stored instead of eliminated from the body, they have the potential to cause future health problems.

Bottom line: Any imbalance in immune function, such as a prolonged exposure to foreign invaders without ridding the body of them, can increase chronic inflammation, decrease the ability to fight off foreign invaders, and increase the potential for autoimmune reactions.

What Do We Mean by "Anti-Inflammation Diet"?

I have found that the best type of diet for many people to adopt to ensure optimal health and healing is an anti-inflammation diet. I learned this diet from my mentor, Dr. Dickson Thom, who teaches at the National College of Naturopathic Medicine (NCNM), where I received my medical degree. I was fortunate to work under Dr. Thom in NCNM's clinic, where I saw amazing benefits from the anti-inflammation diet. We call this diet anti-inflammatory because it eliminates many common allergenic foods that may promote inflammation in the body (see Chapter 2 for a discussion of inflammation). It also reduces intake of pesticides, hormones, and antibiotic residues. The diet is full of whole foods; it eliminates processed foods, sugars, and other man-made foods such as hydrogenated oils, and it encourages ample vegetable intake for essential nutrients. By reducing the intake of toxins and other difficult-to-digest substances, the anti-inflammation diet promotes easier digestion and offers less insult to the body. If the blood and lymph are properly supplied with nutrients and if foods that are difficult to digest or assimilate are eliminated, cellular function—or, in other words, metabolism—improves. Therefore, the body is supported in ways that facilitate cellular regeneration rather than cellular degeneration, which can promote disease.

The anti-inflammation diet that is presented in this book is the most extreme form of the diet. Even partially adopting the diet will promote many positive changes in health. For example, eliminating all white flour, all white sugar, and nonorganic meats while still eating whole wheat, molasses, and organic meats will improve health.

For some individuals and families, making the change to an anti-inflammation diet may be a slow transition. It doesn't have to happen overnight; even gradually adopting the diet will improve health and decrease the chance for future chronic disease. If one already has a chronic disease, a quicker transition to the anti-inflammation diet will make a larger difference in health. For example, an individual with cancer will want to make sacrifices to shift more quickly to the diet; doing so will promote positive changes that will support any cancer treatment the patient is undergoing, whether conventional or otherwise. Again, this diet truly has the potential to cleanse the system enough to make any treatment—allopathic or "alternative"—more effective.

Another thing to remember is that not everyone will react negatively to all of the foods listed in this diet as "foods to avoid." After strictly following the anti-inflammation diet for a certain length of time, reintroducing some of the foods may be acceptable, and if no adverse reactions are noticed during reintroduction, that particular food may be tolerated (but it still shouldn't be consumed daily). How to reintroduce foods is discussed in Chapter 3.

Inflammation: What's the Big Deal?

Researchers are finding more and more evidence linking chronic inflammation with chronic disease. According to an article written by Michael Downey that appeared in the February 2005 issue of the magazine *Better Nutrition,* many inflammatory markers in the body are directly or indirectly related to cardiovascular disease, cancer, Alzheimer's disease, autoimmune diseases, and even asthma. Even healthy cells sometimes mount an immune response against normal cells, resulting in an inflammatory attack on certain tissues such as those found in joints, nerves, and connective tissue. This is how inflammation may be related to autoimmune conditions such as rheumatoid arthritis, multiple sclerosis, lupus, or psoriasis.

What Is Inflammation?

Inflammation is the first response by the immune system to infection or irritation. It presents with the cardinal signs of redness *(*Latin: *rubor)*, heat *(calor)*, swelling *(tumor)*, pain *(dolor)*, and dysfunction of the organs involved. Acute inflammation is needed to help heal acute trauma, abrasions, broken bones, or acute invasion of a foreign substance such as bee venom from a bee sting. The body reacts immediately to acute trauma by increasing substances in the body that stimulate swelling, redness, pain, and heat. These responses are important because they keep the body from doing further damage to the injury or wound by promoting pain and swelling all around the injured area. This causes an individual to be more cautious when moving the affected part. For example, if you break your wrist, the pain and inflammation will force you to protect the wrist from further damage that could occur if you used it or moved it too quickly.

Chronic inflammation is an ongoing, low level of inflammation, invisible to the human eye, that usually occurs as a response to prolonged acute inflammation or repetitive injuries. We are now also finding that chronic inflammation is associated with many diseases. It is unknown how inflammation begins in chronic disease, but there are many theories, some of which are discussed in this chapter.

Chronic inflammation can and will lead to necrosis (tissue destruction) by the inflammatory cells and by certain other agents. The body's healing response depends upon many factors, including persistent infection, the presence of foreign material or other agents that stimulate inflammation (such as latent viruses, bacteria, or parasites), inadequate blood supply, irradiation, and locally applied drugs such as corticosteroids. Other systemic factors include age (the healing process becomes slower and less effective with increasing age); deficiencies in nutrients such as vitamin C, zinc, and protein; chronic food allergies; metabolic diseases such as renal failure or diabetes mellitus; degenerative states associated with malignancies; and systemic drugs such as corticosteroids (these drugs can be used both topically and systemically).

Inflammation, fever, tissue swelling, and allergies are largely controlled by fatty acids called prostaglandins. There are three different families of prostaglandins that serve three different functions in the body:

1. PGE1 helps to reduce allergies, prevents inflammation, increases mucous production in the stomach, decreases blood pressure, improves nerve function, and also helps to promote immune response.

2. PGE2 stimulates the allergy response, promotes inflammation, increases platelet aggregation (when platelets stick to the site of plaque formations along blood vessel walls, leading to the development of localized blood clots, which can further block the flow of blood in the artery), increases smooth-muscle contraction, and suppresses immune function.

3. PGE3 blocks the release of proinflammatory prostaglandins (PGE2), promotes immune function, decreases platelet aggrega-

tion, increases HDL cholesterol (the "good" cholesterol), decreases triglycerides, and inhibits inflammation.

In simple terms, you can think of PGE1 and PGE3 as the "good" prostaglandins and PGE2 as the proinflammatory or "bad" prostaglandin.

As you might expect, certain foods can promote production of certain prostaglandins. Linoleic acid (from safflower oil, sunflower oil and seeds, sesame oil and seeds, and breast milk) is converted into PGE1. Arachidonic acid (from meats, dairy products, and breast milk) is converted into PGE2. Alpha-linolenic acid (from pumpkin seeds, flaxseeds, walnuts, soybeans, and breast milk) is converted into PGE3. Eicosapentaenoic acid (EPA) and docosahexaenoic acid (DHA) can be made by the body from alpha-linolenic acid (ALA). EPA and DHA promote the PGE3 pathway (the "good" pathway) and are found in breast milk and cold-water fish such as salmon, mackerel, sardines, and trout.

Having an understanding of the inflammatory cascade and the way foods can influence inflammatory pathways in the body allows us to understand the importance of nutrient intake on how our body functions as a whole. For example, if we make sure to include plenty of nuts, seeds, and cold-water fish in our diets, we will naturally be inhibiting inflammation. Consuming these foods will increase PGE1 levels, which will in turn inhibit the formation of PGE2, one of the inflammatory prostaglandins.

The bodily enzymes involved in creating prostaglandins and arachidonic acid metabolites are of great importance with regard to the use of anti-inflammatory medication. For example, the important enzyme phospholipase A2 (PLA2) allows arachidonic acid to be released from cell membranes. Arachidonic acid production is the first step in promoting inflammation. Another enzyme, cyclooxygenase, is needed to convert arachidonic acid into PGE2, prostacyclins, and thromboxanes, all of which promote inflammation. (Hint: You can tell a substance is an enzyme if its name ends in –*ase*.) Lipooxygenase is needed to promote the conversion of arachidonic acid into many other inflammation-producing prostaglandins. The cyclooxygenase-1 pathway helps in the formation of the stomach lining, and the cyclooxygenase-2 pathway promotes inflammation. Many anti-inflammation drugs affect both cyclooxygenase pathways, and thus harm the stomach lining. This topic is discussed in more detail later, in the section on the harm in using anti-inflammation drugs for the long term.

Inflammation and Chronic Disease

As mentioned, recent research supports the surprising connection between chronic inflammation and chronic illnesses such as heart disease, autoimmune diseases, cancer, osteoporosis, and more. In February of 2004, *Time* magazine featured a cover article on the connection between certain chronic diseases and inflammation. Let's take a look at the impact of inflammation on a few significant health conditions: heart disease, diabetes, chronic pain (specifically, fibromyalgia), and insomnia.

Heart Disease

Under the umbrella term of "heart disease" we can include conditions such as stroke, atherosclerosis, heart attack, and high blood pressure. The risk factors often checked for heart disease are cholesterol levels, blood pressure, fasting glucose, and, less commonly, C-reactive protein (CRP), homocysteine, lipoprotein A, ferritin, fibrinogen, and a few others. Other risk factors for cardiovascular disease include having a type-A personality, a family history of heart disease, lack of a significant other, sedentary lifestyle, smoking, infection, ischemia, oxidative damage (caused by free radicals), inflammation, and insulin resistance.

Most risk factors for heart disease can stimulate the release of various inflammatory promoters, reactive oxygen species (free radicals), nitric oxide (discussed later), and immune cells as a result of tissue injury. (Again, when we are talking about inflammation in this context, we are talking about inflammation occurring at a cellular level undetected by the human eye.) Micro damage to tissues or repetitive stress on certain tissues can promote tissue injury, which results in an inflammatory reaction of the immune system. In turn, prolonged inflammation puts people at risk for heart disease. This creates a vicious cycle: Many risk factors for heart disease increase inflammation, and, in turn, low-grade inflammation increases risk for heart disease.

The three types of cell that are susceptible to cardiovascular risk factors include epithelial cells, smooth muscle cells, and immune cells.

Epithelial cells line the blood vessels and are responsible for controlling the flow of nutrients, hormones, and immune mediators from cell to cell. They also regulate vascular tone, which affects blood flow through vessels. ("Vascular" means of or relating to the blood vessels or lymph vessels.) Smooth muscle cells help to control constriction and dilation of blood vessels (vasoconstriction and vasodilation), thereby acting as major regulators of blood pressure. Immune cells help to defend and repair the vascular tissue from chemical and biological insult. Any disruption to the homeostasis, or balance, of these cells can contribute to heart disease risk. According to an article published in March 2004 in the journal *Alternative Medicine Review,* chronic inflammation is the most common insult to these three tissue types, resulting in less than optimal functioning of the cardiovascular system.

In response to inflammation that results from tissue injury or exposure to toxic chemicals, epithelial cells produce a variety of molecules that contribute to heart disease risk. These include clotting and coagulation factors, fibrinolysis factors (which can promote abnormal bleeding), prostaglandins, and vascular tone regulators such as nitric oxide. Nitric oxide (NO) is worth mentioning because it plays a major part in the regulation of blood pressure through its vasodilation-promoting capabilities. A prolonged increase in blood sugar, as found in diabetes, will decrease NO, which in turn will lead to increased vasoconstriction and increased blood pressure (hypertension).

During hypertension, some smooth muscle cells may change to more secretory cells instead of the elastic-type cells they are meant to be. Smooth muscle cells are usually elastic in nature to allow adaptation to the varying degree of blood pressure experienced throughout the day. The new, secretory smooth muscle cells can release growth promoters and begin to form a lesion of proliferating secretory smooth muscle cells along the blood vessel. This lesion is clinically significant because as it grows and develops it shows significant cholesterol and lipid deposits that cause the wall to weaken as the cells experience apoptosis (cell death). As this area of cells weakens the vascular wall, it becomes an aneurysm. An aneurysm is a clinically significant cardiovascular risk factor because it has the potential to rupture and cause instant death. In conditions associated with oxidative stress (damage to tissues from free radicals), such as high cholesterol, NO may be elevated but inactive, and therefore unable to promote vasodilation of blood vessels to reduce blood pressure and combat the possibility of aneurysm.

So you might be wondering how all this information is related to an anti-inflammatory diet. Reducing inflammation through diet will reduce inflammatory mediators in the body that cause oxidative damage to cells. Furthermore, reducing inflammation and reducing blood pressure through exercise and diet can decrease many cardiovascular risks. Finally, reducing inflammation can decrease the minor tissue damage that promotes even further inflammation (which triggers a vicious cycle).

How does the anti-inflammation diet accomplish all these things? Excess fat-soluble toxins that we obtain through diet are stored in our fat cells and are transferred to other locations within our body via cholesterol. As we begin to stimulate optimal health through a healthier diet, exercise, and stress reduction, we create a better-functioning immune system and have better detoxification abilities. Exercise helps to eliminate toxins through sweat and breath, and following the anti-inflammatory diet helps to reduce intake of the water-soluble and fat-soluble toxins that are part of the standard American diet, such as pesticide residues, antibiotics, hormones, preservatives, heavy metals, and other chemicals (e.g., artificial colors and flavorings). As our bodies become more efficient and we eat a purer diet—one that eliminates these toxic burdens—cholesterol levels begin to decrease and NO can begin to normalize its function. In addition, healthier lifestyles reduce stress on the body, leading to a reduction in the secretion of stress hormones (discussed in more detail below).

Let me say it again more simply: By decreasing intake of the toxins normally ingested as part of the typical American diet, we can reduce overall inflammation and thereby reduce the load on the cardiovascular and other systems in the body.

Diabetes

Accumulating evidence suggests that chronic low-grade inflammation is also a risk factor for type-II diabetes. A study published by the *American Journal of Clinical Nutrition* in September 2005 reported that a diet high in inflammation-producing foods, such as refined grains, processed meats, and sugars, increased the risk for developing type-II diabetes. The connection between inflammation and diabetes risk was also noted as early as 2001 by the *Journal of the American Medical Association.*

Chronic Pain and Insomnia

Chronic pain, such as that associated with fibromyalgia, can also be related to inflammation. Despite the fact that fibromyalgia is not considered an inflammatory disease, inflammation plays a major role in symptoms associated with the illness. In fibromyalgia patients in particular, disturbed sleep plays a major role in disrupted healing. At night our immune system has the important job of repairing tissues and cleansing the system of foreign antigens, dead cells, and free radicals. When an individual is unable to sleep, such as in chronic pain or fibromyalgia, muscle, blood vessels, and other bodily tissues are not cleansed and repaired adequately for optimal functioning. This creates a situation in which inflammation can occur at a cellular level because tissue is not being repaired correctly, and waste begins to accumulate within the body because the immune system is not adequately eliminating it.

Many fibromyalgia sufferers have low levels of serotonin, a neurochemical that promotes secretion of growth hormone, is responsible for mood, promotes sleep, and increases DHEA levels (DHEA is discussed later). Human growth hormone, which usually increases during sleep, stimulates the growth of new tissue and facilitates carbohydrate metabolism to sustain energy throughout the day. As serotonin levels decrease in fibromyalgia sufferers, growth hormone decreases, insomnia occurs, depression is more likely, and, because of decreased DHEA levels, inflammation is supported. Ninety-five percent of serotonin is produced within the gastrointestinal tract; therefore, it is very important for fibromyalgia sufferers to have a healthy digestive system. Adopting an anti-inflammatory diet decreases the toxic load on the digestive system, promotes the health of the gastrointestinal tract, and decreases the inflammatory response. A better-functioning gastrointestinal tract improves serotonin secretion, which in turn improves sleep and mood. As sleep and mood improve, the immune system is better able to perform detoxification and to repair damaged tissue at night.

When inflammation is reduced via dietary changes, tissues heal adequately, sleep improves, and pain lessens.

Stress and Inflammation

It is extremely important to address the topic of stress due to its direct influence on inflammation. To some degree, our bodies need stress to help us deal with threatening situations. Our bodies respond to stress by secreting various hormones to increase energy. At one time, hundreds of years ago, humans needed that quick rise in adrenaline to help them run from the tiger they encountered in the woods. The daily stress we deal with now arises from stressors such as work, family, deadlines, traffic, accumulation of toxins, and environmental stress, to name a few. Ideally, when stressful events occur, the sympathetic nervous system is activated, stimulating production of a stress hormone called cortisol, which in turn promotes an increase in blood sugar. This increase in blood sugar is designed to supply us with the extra energy needed to run from the tiger, so to say. But in modern industrialized society, there is no tiger to run from, just the stress that increases cortisol and blood sugar. Without the sudden and intense exertion of energy that occurs when we run from the tiger, we are left with elevated levels of cortisol and blood sugar that our body does not need. These days, faced with numerous stressful situations, many people live in a constant state of sympathetic stimulation, resulting in chronically elevated cortisol levels. Prolonged elevated cortisol can lead to thyroid dysfunction, blood sugar abnormalities, weight gain, osteoporosis, high blood pressure, hyperinsulinemia, hypercholesterolemia, and a plethora of other metabolic imbalances.

In addition to increasing cortisol and blood sugar levels, physiological or psychological stress promotes inflammation through the release of certain neuropeptides. (A neuropeptide is a protein that delivers a message within the nervous system.) These inflammatory neuropeptides stimulate a systemic, or whole-body, stress response via stimulation of the sympathetic nervous system and release of stress hormones, of which cortisol is one. (In fact, the release of neuropeptides is what triggers the release of cortisol in the first place. This whole chain of events happens in the blink of an eye.) These stress hormones stimulate release of acute-phase proteins, which are the first promoters of inflammation. One thing to note is that the same neuropeptides that mediate stress also mediate inflammation; therefore it is possible and even likely that stress creates an inflammatory response in the body.

Let's learn a little more about how elevated cortisol and elevated blood sugar can affect health and inflammation. As mentioned, along with prolonged cortisol output comes a prolonged increase in blood sugar, or glucose. High blood sugar over time leads to increased insulin output and to a condition termed insulin resistance. Normally, the job of the hormone insulin is to allow glucose to enter the cell in times of increased energy need or when there is an increase in blood sugar. Insulin resistance occurs when high amounts of insulin are found in the blood along with high amounts of blood sugar, yet the insulin is not being used adequately by the cell's insulin receptors to allow the blood sugar to enter the cell for energy use. Prolonged increased insulin in turn triggers cholesterol production. Therefore, increased stress ultimately leads to increased levels of cholesterol.

Elevated cortisol also contributes to inflammation by increasing levels of interleukin-6 (IL-6), which causes inflammatory reactions and also decreases the part of the immune system responsible for protection from viral and bacterial infections. Over time, elevated levels of cortisol and IL-6 cause a decrease in a very important hormone called DHEA. DHEA, thought of as the immune and antiaging hormone, controls age-related disorders, helps repair and maintain tissues, reduces atherosclerosis, increases insulin sensitivity, controls allergic reactions, and balances the activity of the immune system. One should note that DHEA is available over the counter in health-food stores. However, it should not be taken as a supplement unless the patient's own bodily level of DHEA is found to be low on proper lab tests. Furthermore, supplementation should be directed by a knowledgeable physician.

Negative emotions and lack of supportive relationships significantly affect immune modulation. Several studies have shown that dysregulation of the immune system may play a role in many conditions associated with inflammation, including cardiovascular disease, osteoporosis, arthritis, type-II diabetes, certain cancers, and aging. Negative emotions and prolonged infections have been shown to directly stimulate the proinflammatory cytokines that influence these and many other conditions. According to Robert A. Anderson, who wrote on autoimmune diseases and inflammation in the May 2004 issue of the journal *Townsend Letter for Doctors and Patients,* "Abrasive close personal relationships are seen to provoke persistent immune downregulation." ("Immune downregulation" means a decrease in the ability of the immune system to react efficiently to foreign invaders. It can also mean an overreaction to nonharmful molecules, such as occurs in allergic reactions.) According to Anderson, even negative stressful events from the past that were not processed correctly or resolved increase the risk for cardiovascular disease, metabolic disease, and degenerative diseases such as cancer.

This strongly suggests that treatment of stress-induced conditions requires a holistic approach—one that includes an anti-inflammatory diet, adequate sleep, exercise, and, if indicated, counseling, journaling, affirmations, prayer, *qi gong* (a gentle Chinese healing art that uses a series of focused mind and body exercises), and nutritional supplementation.

The Harm in Chronic Use of Anti-Inflammatory Medication

When someone is in pain, it is common that the individual self-treat with or be prescribed anti-inflammatory medications such as steroid drugs or nonsteroidal anti-inflammatory drugs (also known as NSAIDs). Steroid-based anti-inflammatory drugs inhibit the immune system and interfere with the healing process. The NSAID group includes aspirin, ibuprofen (marketed under the names Motrin and Advil), and naproxen (Aleve). It does not include acetaminophen (Tylenol), which is effective against pain and fever but not against inflammation. Aspirin, ibuprofen, and naproxen inhibit the cyclooxygenase enzymes that promote the production of inflammatory mediators (mentioned above). However, because these drugs are not specific, they also affect the stomach lining, resulting in the possible side effects of ulcers and gastric (stomach) upset. In addition, NSAIDs block the release of the more anti-inflammatory prostaglandins, PGE1 and PGE3, which is contrary to the effect the drug is designed to produce.

Newer anti-inflammatory medications such as rofecoxib (Vioxx) mainly affect the cyclooxygenase-2 pathway; accordingly, they are called COX-2 inhibitors. These drugs are designed to spare the cyclooxygenase pathway that promotes stomach lining health. They help with gastrointestinal side effects, but they have not reduced them completely and are not without their own side effects. And they still promote the lipooxygenase pathway of inflammatory-promoting substances. In September 2004, Vioxx was recalled by the Food and Drug Administration due to its increased risk of cardiovascular events, including heart attack and stroke. Since then, Celebrex, also a COX-2 inhibitor and Vioxx's major competitor, has also raised eyebrows. Its manufacturer, Pfizer Inc., has revealed that it halted a study in December of 2004 linking Celebrex to a "statistically significant" increase in cardiovascular risk. This was at least the second study that showed increased heart problems with the use of Celebrex.

A study published in the *British Medical Journal* in 2005 suggested that regular ingestion of rofecoxib, diclofenac, and ibuprofen significantly increased the risk of having a heart attack. No evidence was found proving that naproxen had any decreased risk for cardiovascular problems. This study and many others in the medical literature offer enough evidence to raise concern about the cardiovascular safety of all NSAID use.

NSAIDs also have noncardiac side-effects such as swelling, rashes, asthma, angioedema (deep swelling beneath the skin), urticaria (hives), anaphylaxis (a potentially life-threatening type of allergic reaction), and many more. It makes sense to adopt a healthy diet that will naturally decrease inflammation rather than relying on the long-term use of anti-inflammatory medications.

CHAPTER 3

❦ ❦ ❦

The Importance of Diet

Adopting a healthy, balanced diet can begin to eliminate many of the problems associated with waste accumulation in the body. It also provides adequate nutrients essential to the body's balanced equilibrium. The role of the digestive system is to bring food in, break it down into useable energy via nutrient absorption, and dispose of wastes that cannot be efficiently used. The higher the quality of food we eat, the more nutrients and energy we obtain from it.

Mitigating the Effects of Toxic Overload

We are exposed daily to both environmental toxins and food byproducts accumulated through diet. As we ingest nonuseable chemicals contained in foods, such as hormones, pesticides, antibiotic residues, and other compounds, our body must work extra hard to digest these foreign substances in addition to obtaining nutrients from the same foods. The liver and kidneys, which are responsible for metabolizing toxic compounds, must work at breaking down toxins from our environment, our food, and our own metabolic processes. The human body is not 100 percent efficient as it performs metabolism. It tends to make wastes, endogenous toxins that need to be processed and excreted from the body. The efficiency with which a person's body excretes these cumulative wastes determines his or her "terrain" (the body's susceptibility to disease due to its biochemical and energetic environment). As this implies, different individuals have different terrains.

In addition to environmental and dietary toxins, pharmaceutical drugs are another source of outside toxins. Again, the liver and kidneys are mainly responsible for catabolizing (breaking down) and excreting these toxins. Finally, in addition to having to metabolize toxins and wastes, the body must be able to digest and break down airborne and food-borne allergens. Does it make sense that we overload our systems by accumulating more toxins? Does it also make sense that reducing dietary toxins can enhance how effectively we eliminate the remaining ones?

Here is an analogy to help you understand the body's capacity for stress, toxins, allergens, and metabolic wastes and how they could relate to your diet. Imagine you have a cup that holds eight fluid ounces. This cup symbolizes your potential toxin and allergen intake. If you fill the cup with six ounces of food allergies, you can take in only two more ounces before the cup overflows and you can no longer deal with the toxins. If you are then exposed to environmental toxins, pollens in the springtime, and pharmaceutical drugs, your cup cannot handle all of the insults to your system. As your cup overflows, you may experience pain, runny nose, postnasal drip, cough, rash, fatigue, and many other symptoms (discussed later in the section on food allergy).

On the other hand, if you remove the six ounces of food allergies, you have an increased ability to take in and process toxins and allergens that cannot be avoided. For example, patients who are extremely allergic to grass and pollen cannot remove all of the grass and pollen from their lives, but they can decrease their food allergies to allow their body to better process grass and pollens.

You Really Are What You Eat

The most important part of my practice in the development of a treatment plan with my patients is diet. You have probably heard the phrase "you are what you eat" a million times throughout your life. Have you ever stopped to think of what the phrase means or why it has become such a popular cliché?

Laws of physics state that every object or being can be broken down into smaller and smaller molecules. The smallest part that makes up any object or being is energy. Because all objects are made of energy, we can deduce that human beings are made wholly of energy. This also means that all food is energy. If we stopped eating energy-giving foods to fuel our body processes, we could not live for very long. That said, doesn't it make sense to pay attention to what we consume each day? The food we eat is the fuel for all bodily processes. If you value your car and want it to run at its optimal level, wouldn't you put the best-quality gas and oil into it? Likewise, if you value your body (and, accordingly, your health and your life), isn't it time to put the best-quality food or "fuel" into it?

Just as different objects have varying energy composition, different foods also have varying energies. We need to pay attention to the quality of food we put into our bodies. Food that is organically grown, is freshly picked, and has spent the least amount of time in transport has the most vitality and therefore will offer you the highest-quality energy and nutrients. The more processing a food undergoes, the more toxins and the less energy and nutrient value it holds. Here's general rule to remember: If you can't tell what a food is by looking at it, don't eat it. For example, white bread is made from wheat, but does it look like wheat? Can you tell it was made from wheat? Then you probably should not eat it.

Eating foods that are locally produced and in season is a great way to ensure good quality and good vitality. Foods that have been dehydrated, boxed for weeks or sometimes months, or canned in aluminum may be devoid of energy and full of preservatives, additives, and possibly dyes. These processed food items may offer a significantly reduced amount of nutrients compared with fresh foods. We can obtain some vital micronutrients (vitamins, minerals, and phytochemicals), which are used to support metabolism and energy, through supplementation, but the macronutrients needed for the body's fuel (carbohydrates, proteins, and fats) can only come from food. Because the food we eat is our only source of fuel, we really are what we eat. Eating food out of cans day after day may leave a person feeling fatigued and devoid of energy, similar to the energy of the food he or she is consuming.

Food Allergies, Food Intolerances, and Inflammation

One vital component of a healthy diet is the elimination of any food allergies or intolerances. Food allergies are becoming increasingly common within our population. I believe the development of food allergies and intolerances is due in part to our nonrotating diet of similar foods. For example, one might eat wheat three or more times a day, in the form of toast for breakfast, a sandwich for lunch, and pasta for dinner.

So, what is a food allergy? Basically, a food allergy is the result of an immune-system reaction to certain food proteins. The immune system stimulates histamine release, resulting in runny nose, watery eyes, and production of throat mucous. More severe reactions can include hives, abdominal cramping, diarrhea, or even anaphylaxis. (A longer list of symptoms of food allergies appears below.)

The immune system's reaction to food allergies can cause inflammatory responses. When someone has an allergy to a certain food, consumption of that food can stimulate production of antibodies that have the potential to bind with the food or to cross-react with normal tissue, resulting in an autoimmune or inflammatory reaction. Any inflammation in the body interferes with and slows down metabolism and the healing response. Furthermore, food allergens often are not digested properly and thus can be another source of "morbid matter" accumulated in the body that must be eliminated via the kidneys, liver, and other organs of detoxification. The anti-inflammation diet eliminates most possible food allergies for most people.

In contrast to a food allergy, a food intolerance is a nonmediated immune reaction. Perhaps an individual lacks the enzymes needed to break down certain foods, such as in milk intolerance (lactose intolerance). Food sensitivities can occur when an individual is unable to eat certain foods, yet does not have an immune reaction to them. I believe another cause of food intolerances or food sensitivities is an imbalance in or a lack of the proper microbial flora that normally line the gastrointestinal tract such as *Lactobacillus acidophilus* and *Lactobacillus bifidus*. The balance of these microorganisms plays a part in how resilient our gastrointestinal tract is.

Symptoms of food allergies and food intolerances often overlap, making it difficult to distinguish the true cause. I am not concerned with why patients cannot eat certain foods; I am concerned with how much better they feel after omitting the offending food from their diets.

Several methods exist to test for food intolerances or allergies. The true gold standard is an elimination and challenge diet. If a person is very diligent, this approach can be an inexpensive and very effective approach to discovering food allergies or intolerances. I reserve this approach to the anti-inflammation diet for individuals with average to good health.

The best way to implement the elimination and challenge diet is to strictly follow the anti-inflammation diet suggested in this book for four weeks. After that time, each food can be introduced individually in its most whole form. For example, to introduce tomatoes, eat one whole tomato after avoiding anything with tomatoes for four weeks; do not eat tomato sauce or tomato soup. After eating the tomato, don't eat any more tomatoes or tomato products for three days because some reactions may be delayed. After three days, assuming you've had no reaction to the tomato, you can probaby assume that tomatoes are a safe food for you. Then you can introduce the next food in its whole form, wait three days, and so on. If you have a reaction immediately, then you can assume the food you introduced is not good for you and that you should avoid it. Since you've already shown a reaction to the recently introduced food, you may introduce the next food without waiting the usual 3 days.

If you have a hard time strictly following the anti-inflammation diet, you may instead eliminate and then reintroduce one food at a time. For example, avoid all dairy products for one month. Then reintroduce it by drinking one glass of milk, and wait up to three days for any reaction. Then eliminate the next food, and so on.

Most people will react to foods in the bodily system where they are most susceptble. For example, if one is prone to migraines, then a migraine may occur; if one is prone to diarrhea or digestive distress, then diarrhea may occur. Reactions are not limited to susceptible systems, however, and can be anything from mild congestion to mood disturbance to severe abdominal cramps. Some reactions may be immediate and some may be delayed; that is why we have individuals wait up to three whole days before introducing the next food.

After following the elimination and challenge diet, one may learn what types of foods he or she reacts to. It has been my experience and observation, however, that for someone with a chronic disease, following the diet the way it is presented will offer the best optimal health. For example, it is recommended that chronically ill patients avoid wheat—even organic whole wheat and even if no reaction is noted during the elmination and challenge phase of the diet—until their health improves and their terrain is treated.

Certain Foods That Contribute to Inflammation

The list of foods to avoid for the anti-inflammation diet includes all wheat products, dairy products, potatoes, tomatoes, corn, sugar, citrus fruits, pork, commercial (nonorganic) eggs, shellfish, peanuts and peanut butter, coffee, alcohol, juice, caffeinated teas, soda, anything containing hydrogenated oils, processed foods, and fried foods. Many of these foods can contribute directly to inflammation. For example, tomatoes and potatoes, which are part of the Solanaceae or nightshade family of vegetables, are known to cause inflammation. Tomatoes and potatoes should definitely be avoided by anyone with arthritis of any kind.

Dairy products are worth mentioning because they tend to be very high in fat. The amount of fat really isn't the problem, though, because the amount of fat-soluble toxins that are stored in the fat becomes the true issue. We know that conventionally raised dairy cows, and consequently dairy products, are bombarded with toxins in the form of pesticide residues on feed and genetically modified soy products in the feed. Many cattle, who are naturally herbivores, are even fed animal protein, which contains its own accumulated toxins and thus in turn further increases the total toxin load in dairy products. As a result, dairy products contribute to the load of toxins that the body's immune system must process and eliminate (or store if the body is under stress and thus unable to eliminate the toxins).

You may be wondering how you are going to obtain the calcium necessary for bone health if you are asked to avoid milk. Isn't avoiding milk especially risky for the development of children's bones? The dairy industry has done an excellent job of marketing the notion that everyone needs to drink milk to keep bones healthy and strong. In fact, there are many nondairy sources of calcium, including fortified soy, rice, oat, almond, and other nut milks.

The body absorbs only about 30 percent of the calcium contained in dairy products. *The Townsend Letter for Doctors and Patients,* in a summary of over twenty different articles, concluded that an allergy to cow's milk is common among adults and children. In fact, intact milk proteins are known to stimulate the secretion of proinflammatory cytokines in susceptible patients, such as those with cow's milk allergy.

In addition, because our standard diet is largely made up of animal proteins (including milk proteins), which are acidic in nature, the body removes calcium from the bones to help balance the pH in the gastrointestinal system.

If one finds they do not react to dairy and want to include it in their diet, I suggest eating only organic dairy products. They don't contain the pesticide residues, hormones, and antibiotic residues regular dairy may contain. That's because the cows are held to higher feeding standards and therefore don't accumulate uneccessary toxins through their diet. Still, even organic dairy products shouldn't be consumed daily.

The best—and an often overlooked—substitute to drinking milk is drinking water. I want my patients to drink half their weight in fluid ounces of filtered water daily. (One cup equals eight fluid ounces. Therefore, a person weighing 140 pounds should drink seventy fluid ounces of water daily, which works out to about nine cups, or a little over two quarts.) Drinking filtered water is important because it reduces the toxin load by filtering out unwanted metals such as aluminum and lead, bacteria, hormones, pesticide residues, industrial polutants, solvents, toxic elements, and other water-soluble toxins. Liquids to consume as part of the anti-inflammation diet include filtered water and herbal teas made with filtered water. All caffeinated beverages and beverages containing sugar are avoided. Juice is avoided because it is a large source of concentrated sugar, even though it is a natural sugar. Ask yourself if you can eat four oranges in one sitting. If the answer is no, then you should not consume an eight-ounce glass of orange juice, which contains the equivalent amount of sugar yet lacks the beneficial fiber content the whole fruit would have.

Alcohol should be avoided because it turns into sugar once in the body. Coffee and other caffeinated beverages are very taxing to the liver due to their toxin load and are taxing to the adrenal glands because of caffeine's effect on cortisol levels. The adrenal glands, located on top of the kidneys, are responsible for maintaining energy, producing sex hormones, balancing blood pressure and blood sugar, and moderating the stress response. If a person's system is already burdened with physiological or psychological stressors, caffeine will exhaust any stress-moderating resources left in the body. Caffeine also has a detrimental effect on weight loss and can cause anxiety, anger, insomnia, and irritability.

Commercial eggs, beef, and pork are included on the list of foods to avoid largely for the same reasons that dairy is to be avoided: because of the toxin content and acidifying nature of the animal protein. Pork and beef are high in arachidonic acid, which, as discussed in Chapter 2, promotes inflammation. Some organic beef is allowed but should be eaten sparingly. Pork, even organic, is not allowed on this diet because of its potential to stimulate an autoimmune reaction and due to its fat quality. Pigs have very similar protein structures to humans; thus, consuming pork can increase the chance of cross-reactions in the immune system. A cross-reaction occurs when the immune system reacts to the pork proteins that are so similar to human proteins, simultaneously triggering an immune response against the body's own cells. In his book *The Maker's Diet,* Jordan Rubin describes pork as an unclean meat; he compares pork with beef based on the complexity of the two animals' digestive systems. Rubin states that meat from cows is a "cleaner" meat than pork because of cows' complex digestion (they have four stomach chambers) and because of what cows eat. Because pigs often live in unclean environments, have noncomplex digestion, and will eat anything, including their own young, he considers them to have lower-quality fats, making them a lower-quality food. Studies have shown that the visible fat content in pork is very high in arachidonic acid compared to beef, though the actual meat of pork is lower in arachidonic acid. The anti-inflammatory diet is developed to nourish the body on all levels. Pork is not allowed on this diet for more than one reason: because of its high levels of arachidonic acid and because of its potential to create immune-system imbalance.

Organic eggs that are free of hormone and pesticide residues and that come from free-range chickens are allowed, but they should not be eaten every day because of their animal-protein content.

Sugar causes many abnormal reactions in the body and should be avoided by all individuals. Sugar depresses the immune system and doesn't offer any nutrients to the diet. Prolonged high-sugar diets contribute to high glucose levels, high insulin levels, and high cholesterol levels, all of which increase heart disease risk, insulin resistance, and diabetes risk.

Shellfish and peanuts are avoided as part of the anti-inflammation diet because many people have allergies to them. Peanuts also grow an aflatoxin on their surface, which has been shown to increase the incidence of cancer in some individuals; peanuts must be processed carefully to avoid production of this substance.

Corn is another common allergen that needs to be avoided. Conventionally grown corn has often undergone a significant amount of genetic engineering and been subjected to heavy bombardment with pesticides.

Wheat is worth discussing, because our standard diet has gone wheat crazy. If you want a good perspective on wheat use in today's diet, ask anyone who has celiac disease, which is a disease of gluten intolerance that results in bowel problems. Think of the typical American family and what they eat on a daily basis. As mentioned above, one might have cereal, toast, or pancakes for breakfast, a sandwich for lunch, and then pasta or pizza for dinner. The typical family may consume wheat three times daily. Today, wheat is not what it was a hundred years ago. Wheat has been greatly genetically modified; furthermore, many nutrients are removed in the refining and processing of wheat. Genetically modifying wheat has increased its gluten content to 90 percent, which is highly irregular. It is possible that the genetic modification of wheat has changed its structure into something our body does not recognize as "safe to pass." In their book *Dangerous Grains,* James Brady and Ron Hoggan describe gluten as a protein that the immune system reacts to pathologically, producing inflammation. Their theory, supported by evidence, is that gluten destroys healthy tissue through molecular mimicry, or cross-reaction. According to an article published in the November 2001 issue of the journal *Annals of Allergy, Asthma, and Immunology,* the substances CRP and IL-6 are increased during acute allergic reactions. Remember that CRP and IL-6 stimulate inflammation. This same reaction can be seen with any food allergy, wheat just being a common example.

Citrus fruits may increase inflammation in the body; they also tend to aggravate arthritis symptoms. It isn't clear why citrus foods trigger inflammatory joint symptoms in some people but not others; however, in many people with rheumatoid arthritis, one or more of the foods to be avoided on this diet will make their condition worse. Again, this doesn't mean that all these foods are necessarily bad for everyone. Just as a bee sting can cause an extreme reaction in one person and not in another, these foods may cause joint pains in some individuals but not others.

Remember that during the elimination and challenge phase of the diet, you may begin to consume these foods again to see if you react to them. For example, if you reintroduce peanuts and do not react to them in a negative way, you can eat them, *but not every day.* (Remember that one of the key features of a healthy diet is variety.) Knowing your food reactions will be helpful in treating and preventing chronic disease. Interestingly, a person may find that they react to nonorganic corn, but not to organic corn.

Finally, besides foods that commonly trigger allergies or sensitivities, other foods that should be avoided are processed foods, foods containing hydrogenated oils, and fried foods. Foods containing hydrogenated oils, including fried foods, stimulate the release of the inflammation-promoting prostaglandins. Any foods that are processed are going to contain large amounts of preservatives, toxins, and dyes, all of which contribute to the body's overall toxic load. In addition, they have often been sitting on shelves for weeks or months before purchase, clearly reducing their level of vital nutrients.

Symptoms of Food Allergies

Symptoms of food allergies or intolerances include headaches, constant clearing of the throat, mucous in the throat, abdominal complaints such as bloating or cramping, irritable bowel syndrome, irritable bowel disease, fatigue, migraines, arthritis, asthma, eczema, psoriasis, most skin complaints, acne, aphthous (mouth) ulcers, sinusitis (inflammation of the sinus cavities, resulting in runny nose and/or congestion), otitis media (ear infection), chronic cough, and chronic allergies to pollens, molds, or other environmental agents. Food allergies may also trigger minor or major mood changes, including depression, anger, hyperactivity, or anxiety.

Other Common Food Allergies

Besides the list of foods to avoid on the anti-inflammation diet, other foods that may trigger allergies or sensitivities include food dyes, especially yellow and red; dried fruit, especially for diabetics due to its concentrated sugar; chocolate, which contains caffeine, and, in the case of milk chocolate, dairy; aspartame (NutraSweet); bananas; meat preservatives (nitrites); monosodium glutamate (MSG); onions; pickled herring; and some vinegars. This diet removes most major food allergens. If you still experience symptoms after following the diet closely, consider removing the rest of these potential irritants from your diet.

⸙ ⸙ ⸙

CHAPTER 4

The Anti-Inflammation Diet

This chapter summarizes how to follow the anti-inflammation diet. The section entitled "The Anti-Inflammation Diet: A Summary," on page 41, is a summary of foods that are allowed and foods to avoid.

The Building Blocks

The basic constituents of any diet include protein, fat, carbohydrate, fiber, vitamins, and minerals. Of these, only protein, fat, and carbohydrate contain calories. (Alcohol also contains calories, but it is not recommended as part of the anti-inflammation diet.) The proportions I suggest for each of these components are listed below:

Macronutrient Percentages for Optimal Health	
Protein	20–30% of total calories
Fat (primarily a balance of essential fatty acids)	20–30% of total calories
Carbohydrate (primarily complex carbohydrates)	40–60% of total calories

Even for people who need or want to lose weight, instead of greatly restricting calories, the anti-inflammation plan allows them to eat a moderate-calorie diet, including healthy snacks throughout the day. The low-fat, low-calorie diet often proposed to achieve weight loss typically ends in a perpetual cycle of weight loss and weight regain. You should not have to greatly restrict calorie intake to lose weight if you are eating the right foods.

Protein

Eating enough good-quality protein at each meal is one of the best ways to maintain appropriate and steady levels of blood sugar, which translate into stabilized energy levels and mood throughout the day. Adult protein intake should equal 45–60 grams per day. Organic sources of protein are best in order to avoid pesticide residues, antibiotics, and hormones. For meat eaters, organic, grass-fed beef is okay, but should be limited to one or two servings weekly. Other meats that are allowed on the diet include free-range, antibiotic-free chicken or turkey (in order to meet USDA standards, poultry cannot be fed hormones), lamb, wild game, and wild fish.

Soy is an excellent source of protein for meat eaters and vegetarians. Sources of fermented soy, such as miso, tempeh, and soy sauce, offer more cancer-fighting antioxidants than nonfermented sources such as soy milk and tofu. Nuts, seeds, and legumes of any type are good sources of protein. Meals that combine grains with legumes make a complete protein. Eggs from free-range, antibiotic-free chickens are a great source of protein. They should be slow cooked, poached, or soft boiled to prevent the oxidation of the egg protein. Avocados have a good amount of protein in addition to healthy fat; they make a great snack for midmorning or afternoon. Are you worried that the avocado contains too much fat? Keep reading.

The Fat Story

At one time or another, we all worried about eating too much fat. That concern should be replaced with the question "Am I eating the *right kind* of fat?" I have a few tips on fat intake that may come in handy as you convert to an anti-inflammatory diet. The body's fat has the potential to store toxins that are not eliminated properly. Therefore, our intake of animal fat should come mostly from organic sources, due to the potential of animals to store toxins in their fat tissue. Furthermore, nonorganic sources of fat may be exposed to more toxins, such as pesticides (which can come from both animal and plant sources of fat), antibiotics, hormones, and other such compounds.

Three Types of Fat

Fat intake is extremely important for our bodies. We need some fat in our diet to maintain vital body functions, to incorporate into cell membranes, and to inhibit excessive fat storage. Again, instead of worrying so much about the *amount* of fat we eat, we need to concentrate more on the *type* of fat we take in. There are three different types of fats:

saturated, monounsaturated, and polyunsaturated. Saturated fats mostly come from dairy products, red meats, poultry, and many processed foods. Saturated fats also occur in coconut oil and palm oil. We need a certain amount of saturated fat in our diets to produce cholesterol, which is an important component of cell membranes as well as acting as a precursor to all of the steroid hormones (e.g., pregnenolone, progesterone, cortisol, and aldosterone), each of which has a distinct function within the body. For example, progesterone and pregnenolone have antioxidant, antiseizure, antispasm, anticlotting, anticancer, promemory, and promyelination functions, and are helpful in regulating women's menstrual cycles.

Monounsaturated fat, found in oils such as canola and olive oil and also in avocados, has been called the "good fat," which in part is true. Eating sufficient amounts of monounsaturated fat has been shown to decrease LDL cholesterol, the "bad" cholesterol.

Let's talk for a moment about canola oil, which is currently being touted as a "healthy" oil. Canola oil, which comes from the seed of the rape plant (it is known as rapeseed oil in other countries), is poisonous to many living things. It is used as an insect repellent and was the source of the chemical warfare agent mustard gas, which was banned after it was shown to blister the lungs and skin of many soldiers. The name "canola" comes from the fact that rapeseed oil was modified in a Canadian laboratory into a lower-acid oil presumed safe for human consumption (the word "canola" stands for Canadian oil low acid). The Canadian government paid the U.S. Food and Drug Administration (FDA) a large sum of money to have canola oil placed on the "Generally Recognized as Safe" (GRAS) list. However, studies of the effects of canola oil on lab animals show problems related to the heart, adrenals, kidneys, and thyroid. No human studies were performed before canola oil was widely promoted in the United States.

When baking, I used to use organic butter and canola oil. I have now switched for all of my baking to a blend of organic butter and organic coconut oil. Coconut oil and butter, because they are saturated fats, are stable in high temperatures and remain stable for the extended time needed for baking. The damage done by oxidation of fats usually occurs when heating a relatively unstable fat such as a monounsaturated or polyunsaturated fat. Using a monounsaturated fat such as canola oil in baking or cooking leaves the body more susceptible to oxidative damage. An unsaturated fat, when heated, has the potential to convert into a trans fatty acid, which the body is unable to metabolize. (Trans fatty acids are discussed in more detail below.)

Oxidative damage to the body increases the risk of forming atherosclerotic plagues in the arteries, which in turn increase the risk for heart disease. Because of the increased risk of oxidative damage that occurs when heating a monounsaturated fat to high temperatures, it is important to make sure you avoid heating olive oil too high when cooking with it. If you are stir-frying or otherwise cooking at an elevated temperature, use coconut oil instead. Because coconut oil is a shorter-chain saturated fat, it is more easily metabolized by the body than many other saturated fats. I have used coconut oil in place of olive oil for stir-fries, baking, and prolonged heating with great results and no difference in taste. Coconut oil is solid at room temperature. Studies reveal that coconut oil stored at room temperature for over one year still shows no evidence of rancidity. Studies have also suggested that using coconut oil regularly may reduce total cholesterol levels. Individuals living in regions where coconut oil is eaten regularly have generally lower cholesterol levels than individuals living in the United States who eat the typical American diet of processed foods and processed oils.

Essential Fatty Acids

Polyunsaturated fats are made up of omega fatty acids. Omega-3 and omega-6 fatty acids are the essential fatty acids. They are termed "essential" because the human body is unable to produce them and therefore we must obtain them through diet. In ancient times the fat content of our diet was more balanced between omega-3 fats and omega-6 fats. Since our diet has changed to include more processed and refined foods, the ratio has become significantly disproportionate. We typically consume twenty to twenty-five times more omega-6 than omega-3 fatty acids. In addition, the fat content of our diets consists largely of saturated and hydrogenated fats (hydrogenated fats are discussed later).

Omega-6 fatty acids include oils such as borage oil and evening primrose oil. Most nuts and seeds contain a combination of both types of oils. Omega-3 fatty acids come from cold-water fish such as salmon, tuna, sardines, halibut, and mackerel, as well as flaxseeds, other seeds, some nuts, and some legumes. Omega-3 fatty acids should be consumed at least three to four times per week. Some symptoms associated with a deficiency of omega-3 fatty acids are severe allergies, inflammatory conditions, dry hair and skin, brittle nails, eczema or other skin rashes, and bumps on the backs of the upper arms (keratosis pilaris). Essential fatty acids help to promote a healthier nervous system, including improved brain function, mood, memory, and nerve conduction; help improve lipid profiles; are antiatherosclerotic; help promote healthy skin; and support proper immune function.

Ways to supplement include consuming flaxseed oil, cod liver oil, evening primrose oil, essential fatty acid capsules, freshly ground flaxseeds, pumpkin seeds, sesame seeds, and sunflower seeds. The oils should not be heated before ingesting. Flaxseeds should be ground rather than used whole because grinding them releases their fatty acids. Eating them whole gives you the fiber benefits but less of the fatty acid content. Grinding flaxseeds fresh daily (in a clean coffee grinder) is important because after a few days the oil content of ground seeds is no longer fresh.

Hydrogenated Oils

Hydrogenated oils, which are manufactured to make liquid oils like canola and soybean oil solid at room temperature in order to give baked goods a longer shelf life, are used in approximately forty thousand food products in the United States, according to Margo Wootan at the Center for Science in the Public Interest. Hydrogenated oils (or partially hydrogenated oils) are contained in General Mills Total Bran Flakes, Ritz Crackers, Rold Gold Pretzels, and Nabisco Graham Crackers. They are even used in seemingly innocuous foods like some breads, margarines, and peanut butter, and also in some low-fat "health foods," like Tiger's Milk energy bars. Hydrogenated oils give packaged cookies and crackers the crispy, buttery taste we have come to expect, and most of the processed foods we eat wouldn't taste the same without them.

Hydrogenated oils are manmade fats that the body has a limited ability to recognize, break down, or utilize. Why are they called "hydrogenated"? Certain oils are processed in a way that adds hydrogen atoms to their chemical structure. This "hydrogenation" process allows scientists to harden oils that are normally liquid at room temperature to make margarine and other butter alternatives. The new fat is also called a "trans fatty acid" or a "trans fat." According to the *Journal of Clinical Nutrition,* studies from Harvard University in 2004 revealed that trans fats may increase levels of inflammation in the body. The same researchers also found that trans fats may worsen the inflammation already present in people with heart failure.

Trans fats, when used to replace healthy fats in the diet, could render several of the body's vital systems defective. If we accumulate enough of these "indigestible fats" to overload the system, the risk for cancer and other noncommunicable diseases could potentially increase.

According to Donald Yance, author of *Herbal Medicine, Healing, and Cancer,* in 1977 the World Health Organization sent out an alert to all nations stating that continuing to use hydrogenated fats would cause detrimental health effects in the future. Do you know that not one nation listened? Today, chronic diseases—such as cancer, diabetes, and other cardiovascular diseases (primarily heart disease and stroke)— are among the most prevalent, costly, and preventable of all health problems. Seven of every 10 Americans who die each year, die of a chronic disease.

I am not saying that hydrogenated oils are the only cause of chronic disease; I am saying that they play a part in the many lifestyle components that seem to have increased our risk for chronic conditions. What we do know is that hydrogenated oils promote inflammation by stimulating the increase of inflammation-promoting prostaglandins, as mentioned earlier.

Also as mentioned earlier, any oils or fats that are cooked at very high temperatures convert to trans fats. Be cautious when stir-frying that you avoid using a temperature that is too high. If the oil begins smoking, the heat is too high. Also, the oil content in anything that is deep fried and then left to sit in the fryer, such as in fast food restaurants, becomes a trans fatty acid and should be avoided. Finally, in order to avoid changing the fat configuration of eggs, it is best to cook them slowly with low heat. According to *Every Woman's Book,* by Paavo Airola, N.D., use the following procedure to prepare scrambled eggs: Separate them, placing the yolks to the side. The whites are to be poached, removed from the heat, and added to the raw yolks. Scramble the whites and yolks briefly before serving.

Carbohydrates

Eat mostly complex carbohydrates that are unprocessed, unrefined, and as close to their whole, natural state as possible. Whole oats, whole rye, millet, whole-wheat pasta, bulgur, barley, legumes (such as pinto beans, lentils, navy beans, lima beans, split peas), fresh vegetables, brown rice, and sweet potatoes are good sources of complex carbohydrates. Whole grains are a great source of B vitamins, and legumes eaten with grains are a great source of complete protein. Dark-green, leafy vegetables are an excellent source of calcium and zinc.

Simple carbohydrates, such as those found in refined, processed, and sweetened foods, should be limited or excluded from the diet. They include sources of sugars, fruits, white flour, pastries, doughnuts, cookies, soda pop, caffeinated beverages, white rice, cereals made with sugar or enriched grains, and other products whose ingredient list says "wheat" but does not include the word "whole" in front of it. Simple carbohydrates raise blood sugar levels quickly and cause the body to increase insulin production, which triggers cholesterol synthesis. Therefore, increased insulin output caused by excessive amounts of sugar in the diet increases cholesterol levels, as well as promoting fat production and fat storage. Simply put, simple carbohydrates exacerbate diabetes, obesity, high cholesterol, and poor lipid profiles.

Fiber

Fiber is not a specific nutrient, but it is very important for digestive health. It acts as a bulking agent to help pass the stool through the intestine. Inadequate amounts of fiber in the diet can lead to digestive complaints such as constipation and, less often, diarrhea. Fiber also helps to increase transit time to insure that more toxins aren't absorbed into the bloodstream because the stool has remained in the rectum for an extended period of time. Fiber in the diet can help fend off food allergies, improve the body's ability to utilize nutrients, and keep the whole digestive tract clean. The National Institutes of Health recommends that adults consume 35 grams of fiber per day. I recommend at least that much, but 40–50 grams is even better.

Fiber can be found in fresh vegetables, fruits, legumes, and grains. Ground flaxseeds can be a great source of fiber, protein, and omega-3 essential fatty acids. I suggest eating two tablespoons of freshly ground flaxseeds daily. Store your seeds in a jar in the refrigerator, pull the jar out every morning, measure two tablespoons into a clean coffee grinder, grind, and then add them to your cereal or a salad, or mix them with a little water and drink them. Another creative way to get flaxseeds into your diet is to roll them into a ball with almond butter and honey (see the recipe for Sun Candies in the section "Sweet Things").

Eat More of These Foods

In the last chapter I listed foods to avoid when following the anti-inflammation diet. Now let's discuss items that are positive to include in the diet because they help to decrease inflammation. Here's a list:

* Essential fatty acids found in cold-water, oily fish such as salmon, mackerel, tuna (limit to 2 servings per month), sardines, halibut; also, oils extracted from these fish

* Pineapple, because of its content of bromelain, which decreases inflammation

* Fruits and vegetables, except those listed in the table below

* Garlic, ginger, and turmeric

* Most nuts and seeds, except peanuts

* Flaxseed oil; olive oil if not heated too high

* Filtered water, in the amount of half of your body weight in fluid ounces daily (one cup equals eight fluid ounces)

The Anti-Inflammation Diet: A Summary

Posting a copy of this summary on the refrigerator has been helpful for many of my patients.

* Try to eat only organically grown foods to decrease your exposure to pesticides. Furthermore, according to a fact sheet produced by The Soil Association of the U.K. that summarizes an article by James Cleeton appearing in the journal *Coronary and Diabetic Care in the UK* in 2004, organic foods reduce the amount of toxic chemicals ingested, are not genetically modified, reduce the amount of food additives and colorings, and increase the amount of beneficial vitamins, minerals, EFAs, and

antioxidants consumed, which are used by the body to fight cancer and chronic disease.

* There is no preset restriction on the amount of food you can eat, and there is no need to count calories. Pay attention to your body's own satiety signals. Eat when you're hungry, and stop eating when you're satisfied.

* The specific foods listed below are only *examples* of foods to eat, so experiment.

* Try to plan meals with approximately the following caloric composition: 40 percent carbohydrates, 30 percent protein, and 30 percent healthy fats.

* Do not eat any one food more than five times per week.

* Plan your meals ahead of time.

* Try to find at least ten recipes from this book that you enjoy.

Food Category	Foods to Eat	Foods to Avoid
Vegetables: Vegetables are classified progressively according to carbohydrate content. Those in group 1 have the least amount of carbohydrate; those in group 4 have the most. Eat mostly lower-carbohydrate vegetables (those in groups 1 and 2).	*Group 1:* Asparagus, bean sprouts, beet greens, broccoli, red and green cabbage, cauliflower, celery, Swiss chard, cucumber, endive, lettuce (green, red, romaine, mixed greens), mustard and dandelion greens, radishes, spinach, and watercress	Tomatoes; potatoes
Lightly steaming vegetables improves the utilization or availability of the nutrients, allowing the GI mucosa to repair itself. Minimize your intake of raw vegetables, except in salads. Include at least 1–2 servings of green vegetables per day, though even more is preferred.	*Group 2:* String beans, beets, bok choy, brussels sprouts, chives, collards, eggplant, kale, kohlrabi, leeks, onion, parsley, red pepper, pumpkin, rutabagas, turnips, and zucchini	
	Group 3: Artichokes, parsnips, green peas, winter squash, carrots	
	Group 4: Yams and sweet potatoes	

Food Category	Foods to Eat	Foods to Avoid
Grains: Include 1–2 cups of cooked grains per day unless you desire to lose weight.	Amaranth, spelt, barley, buckwheat, millet, oatmeal, quinoa, basmati or brown rice, rye, and teff Rice crackers and Wasa brand rye crackers are also okay.	All wheat products, including breads, cereals, whole-wheat flour, white flour, and pasta that is made from wheat
Legumes: Soak legumes overnight and cook them slowly the next day.	Split peas, lentils, kidney beans, pinto beans, black beans, garbanzo beans, fermented soybeans (tempeh or miso), mung beans, and adzuki beans	Tofu can cause reactions in some people. Experiment with both including it and eliminating it from the diet.
Seafood: Wild (versus farmed) deep-sea, cold-water fish are an excellent source of essential fatty acids and should be eaten 3–4 times per week. Poach, bake, or broil the fish.	Wild salmon, cod, haddock, halibut, mackerel, sardines, tuna, trout, and summer flounder	Shellfish, including shrimp, crab, lobster, clams, and mussels
Meat: Eating protein with every meal helps to regulate and maintain steady blood sugar and energy levels.	Meat only (i.e., not the skin) of organic, free-range chicken and turkey Wild game, venison, and elk Organic, free-range lamb and buffalo	Pork Conventionally raised beef (small amounts of organic, grass-fed beef are okay)
Spices and herbs	Use any favorite herbs and spices to enhance the flavor of your food.	
Fruits: Eat only 1–2 servings of any fruit per day. Try to eat mostly fruits from the lower-carbohydrate categories (Groups 1 and 2).	*Group 1:* Cantaloupe, rhubarb, melons, strawberries *Group 2:* Apricots, blackberries, cranberries, papayas, peaches, plums, raspberries, kiwis *Group 3:* Apples, blueberries, cherries, grapes, pears, pineapples, pomegranates *Group 4:* Bananas, figs, prunes	Citrus fruits (lemon is okay) Limit your intake of dried fruits, and eliminate them if you are diabetic.
Sweeteners: Use sweeteners only occasionally	Pure maple syrup, brown rice syrup, raw honey, agave syrup, stevia	Absolutely no sugar, NutraSweet, or any other sweetener is allowed.

Food Category	Foods to Eat	Foods to Avoid
Butter and oils: Mix 1 pound organic butter with 1 cup extra-virgin olive oil to use as a spread. Store in refrigerator.	A small amount of organic butter is okay. Use olive oil for cooking, coconut oil for baking, and nut or seed oils for salads.	Hydrogenated oils, partially hydrogenated oils (trans fats) Avoid overheating oils, which in the process can convert to trans fats.
Eggs and dairy products	Organic eggs	Dairy products, including yogurt, cheese, and animal milks Commercial eggs
Nuts and seeds: Eat them raw or grind and add them to steamed vegetables, cooked grains, salads, cereals, etc.	Flax, pumpkin, sesame, sunflower seeds Most nuts and nut butters	Peanuts and peanut butter
Beverages	Minimum of ½ your weight in fluid ounces per day of filtered water Small amount of rice, oat, almond, or soy milk Herbal teas (substitute for coffee and juice)	Coffee, soda, juice, caffeinated teas, alcohol
Miscellaneous		Corn products Processed foods Fried foods

Lifestyle Choices

Our current home and work habits often fail to allow for a regular meal schedule. People's busy lives may prevent their caloric intake from being evenly distributed throughout the day. Dinner, often eaten very late and thus soon followed by several hours of sleep, is typically people's biggest meal. When we should be digesting the food we just ate, we are often sleeping, and during sleep our metabolic function is sluggish.

Americans' fast-paced lives have also supported on-the-go meals such as fast food and prepared meals, and quick blood-sugar fixes such as candy bars and other processed sweets. According to the book *Fast Food Nation,* by Eric Schlosser, fast food accounts for 40 percent of Americans' dietary intake. Researchers from Brigham and Women's Hospital, a teaching affiliate of Harvard Medical School, conducted a study published in the *International Journal of Cancer* in 2006, revealing that preschoolers who regularly ate French fries had an increased risk for breast cancer. In fact, researcher Dr. Karin Michels and colleagues estimated that a woman's risk of breast cancer in later life increased by 27 percent for each additional serving of French fries per week that she ate as a preschooler. These foods are not the best-quality fuel we can feed to our bodily processes.

Our children have an even greater need for energy-giving foods to promote growth and good health. My views of childhood development and nutrition were enhanced and enlightened by attending a seminar in Portland, Oregon, offered by Dr. Gerard Gueniot, a medical doctor from France. As he states, "children under the age of four do not have the same digestive capability as adults do; therefore it is a crime to be feeding these toxic-filled, processed foods to young children." Children (as well as adults) benefit immensely from adopting a healthy daily diet of vegetables, fruits, whole grains, nuts, seeds, and a moderate amount of high-quality protein. Parents need to set the example for children, and aware individuals need to set the example for the rest of society. People who understand the importance of a healthy, balanced diet are responsible for teaching the rest of the population how important nutrients are in promoting health and fighting disease. What better way to teach people than by example? It is especially important to share our knowledge with the children who are around us. After all, they are the next leaders of our world.

Mealtime Recommendations

Here are my suggestions for enhancing the quality of mealtimes. Spend time with your food. Do not do anything else such as watching TV, driving, or talking on the phone. Have a quiet, relaxed atmosphere in which to enjoy your food. Reflect upon the energy the food holds and what it is giving to you. Do not drink anything while eating. If you must have something, it should be limited to small sips of water.

Proper chewing is an important part of digestion and should be something that you concentrate on doing during each meal. If you fail to chew your food thoroughly, digestion is not properly initiated and your body will less adequately absorb important nutrients. I suggest that people chew their food at least nineteen times before swallowing.

This ensures that a nearly liquidified product will enter the stomach for easier absorption.

It is best to eat your meals at regularly scheduled times. Eating at the same times each day will establish a pattern with your endocrine system, helping to facilitate digestion at those times. Do not eat late at night, when your metabolism is getting ready to rest.

Make sure to eat breakfast. Eating a whole-grain breakfast has been related to a 15 percent reduction in the risk for insulin resistance, a syndrome that can lead to type-II diabetes, weight gain, and cardiovascular complications. Refined "kid's" cereals, breads, pastries, and other carbohydrates typically consumed for breakfast will not have the same effect as whole grains. Eating all meals, starting with breakfast, is important to maintaining a revved-up metabolism throughout the day.

A Few More Suggestions

The purpose of this book is to act as a guide to help you learn to cook healthily. It is not intended to be something you have to use each time you cook. My goal is to teach you how to cook, how to learn from your mistakes, how to experiment, and how to learn from those positive accidents that create new meal ideas. Learning to cook is a process of developing your skills. Put a little pizzazz into your meals. Experiment. Be creative. You can use many of the recipes in this book as a template for even greater meals. If you are lacking one or two ingredients, replace them with something you do have. I have included some simple beginning recipes that can go in many different directions. Don't be afraid to mix vegetables or grains with fruit. Adding a small amount of fruit to a green salad can be a refreshing treat on a summer day.

Experiment with herbs and spices. Each week, choose one new seasoning to play with and learn about. Look up its medicinal properties, and be appreciative for its actions in your body. If you don't feel comfortable experimenting with a recipe in the beginning, then follow the directions exactly and think of how you can make it better the next time. Maybe you like more spice or less spice. Cook to please yourself and, of course, anyone else dining with you.

Cooking healthily can take very little time. Although it is a passion of mine to spend hours in the kitchen cutting vegetables and preparing meals, I also have a busy health-care practice, a husband, and a child to tend to. I am no stranger to "quick meals." Thinking ahead of time helps to make even quick meals nutritious and full of life-giving energy. One time-saving hint is to chop vegetables ahead of time—for example, when you get home from the grocery store. If I know that I will be preparing a few different meals that require chopped onion, I will chop two to three onions and store them in an airtight container until I need them.

As with anything, the more you practice, the better cook you will become. Host weekly or monthly potlucks with friends and family to share and learn recipes. Most of my inspiration for cooking has come from my fellow naturopathic colleagues, including my husband. It is important to have support when changing your diet. Get your family members and friends involved, and most of all, have fun.

❧ ❧ ❧

How to Use This Book

I have tried to make this book very easy to use and the recipes easy to follow. Some recipes may include foods that are allergenic for some individuals, but I have made suggestions for how to substitute other foods in those cases. In fact, nearly every recipe offers ideas for substitutions. In addition, a substitutions table appears in the Appendix that will help you when you want to do some experimenting with ingredients.

Besides offering substitution ideas, each recipe contains a tidbit of health information about the recipe or about one of the ingredients. It is a bonus to be able to know how you are improving your health each time you prepare a recipe. Most of the recipes are easy to follow and even appetizing to most kids. The key for children is introducing them to healthful ways of eating when they're young and keeping them away from processed foods and sugars. There is always a substitute for sugary items.

Converting Yourself and Your Family

As you have probably learned, children, and even some adults, can be finicky eaters. Drastically changing your family's diet can be difficult and can meet with resistance. In order to sneak healthy foods to family members, you must master the art of adding valuable, life-sustaining nutrients to each meal. It can be as simple as adding flaxseeds and other types of seeds to baked goods. Vegetables should be eaten regularly, so if you're the primary meal-preparer in your household, make it a goal to "slip them in" as often as possible. According to one of my favorite cookbooks, Jane Kinderlehrer's *Confessions of a Sneaky Organic Cook,* the key to sneaky cookery is having a mini food processor or blender. I would add to that list a coffee grinder as well.

Here are some examples of how to include vegetables without your family knowing it. Steam some vegetables, "for yourself" if anyone asks, and purée them in the blender when no one is looking. Add the puréed vegetables to your meal by using them to thicken and flavor many sauces, soups, salad dressings, chicken or tuna salads, veggie burgers, turkey burgers, meatballs, meatloaf, and more. You can add grated zucchini or carrots to cookies, muffins, or pancake batter. Make sure all of your soups contain vegetables. If your younger kids won't eat them, purée them first and then add them to the soup. Be creative and experiment, but don't overdo it at first or your family will find out that what they're eating is not just sauce or soup or whatever.

Be Prepared

An important aspect of being a sneaky cook is being prepared. During the weekend, plan meals for the whole week if you can. Know when you and your children like to snack, and at those times have ready-made snacks to put out on the end tables or on the kitchen counter. As your kids come into the house looking for a snack, they will naturally graze first on what is available and in sight. Some of my favorite snacks are celery or apples with almond butter, nuts, seeds, fruit cut into easy-to-eat pieces, and rice crackers with avocado or hummus.

Modifying Recipes

Learning how to change recipes is another important part of anti-inflammatory cooking. Acquiring this skill takes a little practice, but once you have mastered it you can modify almost any recipe (refer to the Appendix for substitution ideas).

The typical cookie recipe looks somewhat like this:

3 cups white flour

3/4 cup brown sugar

3/4 cup white sugar

2 eggs

1 cup butter or shortening

1/2 teaspoon salt

1/2 teaspoon baking soda

1 bag chocolate chips

With a little practice it becomes easy to substitute alternate flours and sweeteners. Your new recipe may look something like this:

1½ cups spelt flour

1½ cups rice or garbanzo flour

¾ cup honey

½ cup organic butter

½ teaspoon sea salt

½ teaspoon aluminum-free baking soda

2 organic eggs (or 1 mashed banana with 3 tablespoons ground flaxseeds soaked in ¼ cup water overnight)

1 cup nuts and/or seeds

½ cup cut-up fruit such as apricots or apples

If you look at the new recipe, you'll see that we have cut the butter and sugar in half and have added some nuts, seeds, and fruit instead of chocolate chips. You may increase the amount of butter slightly if you want your cookie to flatten more. This new cookie contains some protein to curb the appetite and stabilize blood sugar. We won't have to eat as many of these cookies to fill up as we would the cookies from the old recipe. If you are craving chocolate, you can add carob powder in place of the chocolate chips. Adding cinnamon will help maintain balanced blood glucose. Or you can add coconut. See how fun this can be? You can experiment with adding many new ingredients. I add zucchini to my cookies, and it keeps them moist for weeks, in which case, they should be refrigerated.

Helpful Items to Have in the Kitchen

You don't have to go to the grocery store and purchase everything on this list. Think of it as a template for things you may want to keep on hand to be able to follow many of the recipes in this book.

1. Extra-virgin, cold-pressed olive oil (purchase only oils that have been refined without using heat—e.g., "cold-pressed," "expeller-pressed"—to avoid the possibility of their having been converted into trans fats through the heating process)

2. Organic coconut oil for baking

3. Onions

4. Garlic
5. Raw honey or agave syrup
6. Brown rice syrup
7. Pure maple syrup
8. Nonwheat flours such as spelt, oat, quinoa, rye, barley, rice
9. Lemons
10. Rice vinegar, balsamic vinegar, tarragon vinegar, organic apple cider vinegar
11. Dried herbs and spices, e.g., basil, oregano, thyme, garlic powder, sea salt, black pepper, cumin, curry, cinnamon, turmeric, mustard seeds, mustard powder, nutmeg, carob powder, and any others you like
12. Filtered water
13. Nuts and seeds
14. Fresh fruits
15. Fresh vegetables
16. Brown rice, quinoa, oats, amaranth, other grains
17. Almond butter
18. Pure maple syrup
19. Milk substitutes such as rice milk, oat milk, soy milk, almond milk
20. Beans and legumes, canned or dried
21. Large skillet to stir-fry vegetables
22. Large pot for sauces and soups
23. Two-quart saucepan for cooking rice and other grains
24. Laughter, a good appetite, and the courage to discover new tastes!

Sample Menus

The two tables below outline sample eating plans for the summer and winter months respectively. They are intended only as examples; inclusion in one table or the other does not mean that a particular food should only be eaten in that specific season. Suggestions for physical activity are also included.

Sample Anti-Inflammatory Menus for the Summer Months

	Monday	Tuesday	Wednesday	Thursday	Friday	Saturday	Sunday
Breakfast	Breakfast Smoothie	Protein Power Breakfast	Breakfast Smoothie	2 soft-boiled eggs; 1 serving of fruit	Granola with milk substitute; 1 serving of fruit	Broccoli and Olive Frittata	Wheat-Free Pancakes
Midmorning snack	Can of salmon with rice crackers	Rice protein bar	Nuts and seeds	Celery with almond butter	Apples with almond butter	Guacamole with rice crackers	Hummus with raw vegetables
Lunch	Beet and Bean Salad (made the night before)	Green salad with avocado and nuts	Raw Beet Soup (made the night before)	Quinoa Vegetable Salad (made the night before)	Carrot Beet Salad (made the night before)	Tangy Coconut Soup; brown rice	Cold Asian Noodles with Smoked Salmon
Afternoon snack	Nuts and seeds	1–2 soft-boiled eggs	Baba Ghanoush with rice crackers	Avocado Tuna Salad	Nuts and seeds	Sun Candies	1 slice of The All-Forgiving Banana Bread
Dinner	Cucumber Salad; Baked Tofu; Steamed Vegetables	10-Minute Avocado Soup; Fresh green salad	Turkey Meatloaf; Spicy Honey Lemon Salad with dandelion greens	Chicken Curry Made Simple (chicken baked the night before)	Strawberry Spinach Salad with Blackened Salmon	Seared Tuna over Raw Vegetables	Grilled chicken, turkey, or fish with Vegetable Marinade for Grilling

Include these things daily:

Seeds	2 tablespoons ground flaxseeds
Water	½ your weight in fl. oz. per day (do not drink while eating)
Movement	30–45 minutes walking, exercising, moving outdoors

Sample Anti-Inflammatory Menus for the Winter Months

	Monday	Tuesday	Wednesday	Thursday	Friday	Saturday	Sunday
Breakfast	Quickest Oatmeal You'll Ever Eat	Protein Power Breakfast	Quickest Oatmeal with frozen berries and honey	Granola with milk substitute; 1 serving of fruit	Quickest Oatmeal, any way you like it	Mexican Morning Eggs	Tofu Scramble
Midmorning snack	Nuts and seeds	Seeds; 1 serving of fruit	Rice protein bar	Can of salmon with rice crackers	2 soft-boiled eggs	Hummus with celery sticks	Sun Candies
Lunch	Avocado Tuna Salad over bed of fresh greens	Leftover Veggie Burgers (made the night before from leftovers)	Curry Chicken Salad with crackers or salad greens (chicken baked the night before)	Mexican Salad (make the dressing the night before)	Curried Quinoa Salad (made the night before)	Cream of Carrot and Ginger Soup	Stuffed Mushrooms; Small green salad
Afternoon snack	Almond butter with celery	2 soft-boiled eggs	Almond butter with apples	Nuts and seeds	Avocado with rice crackers	1 slice of Zucchini Bread	Italian Carrot Salad
Dinner	Simple Stir Fry with your favorite grain	Stuffed Chicken Breast with "Peanut" Curry Sauce; Scrumptious Green Beans	Blackened Salmon; Tasty Lemon Vinaigrette Salad	Nutty Onion Soup; Steamed Vegetables	Greek night: Barbecued Kafta, Not-So-Greek Salad, Hummus, and fresh vegetables or rice crackers	Winter Soup; Rice crackers	Breaded Red Snapper with Mango Salsa; Garlic Bean Salad; Sweet Potato "Fries"

Include these things daily:

Seeds	2 tablespoons ground flaxseeds
Water	½ your weight in fl. oz. per day (do not drink while eating)
Movement	30–45 minutes walking, exercising, moving outdoors

∽ ∽ ∽

"The doctor of the future will give no medication, but will interest his patients in the care of the human frame, diet and in the cause and prevention of disease."

THOMAS A. EDISON

∽ ∽ ∽

Volume Equivalents

1½ teaspoons = ½ tablespoon

1 tablespoon = 3 teaspoons

2 tablespoons = 1 ounce = ⅛ cup

1 cup = 8 ounces (16 tablespoons)

1 pint = 2 cups = 16 ounces

1 quart = 2 pints = 4 cups = 32 ounces

1 U.S. gallon = 4 quarts = 16 cups = 128 ounces

Converting U.S. to Metric Measurements

1 ounce = 30 grams

1 teaspoon = 4.9 milliliters

1 cup (16 tablespoons/8 ounces) = 240 milliliters

4 quarts (1 U.S. gallon/128 ounces) = 3.8 liters

teaspoons x 4.93 = milliliters (ml)

tablespoons x 14.79 = milliliters

fluid ounces x 29.57 = milliliters

cups x 236.59 = milliliters

pints x 473.18 = milliliters

quarts x 946.36 = milliliters

U.S. gallons x 3.785 = liters

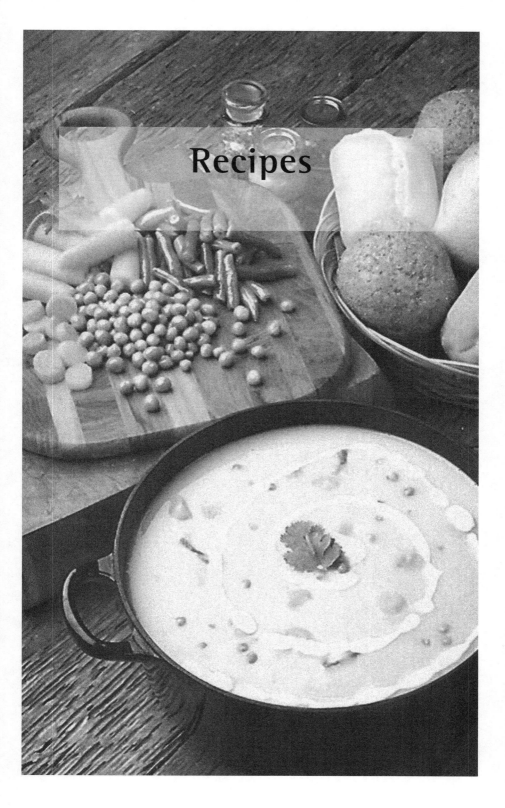

Recipes

Appetizers, Side Dishes, Seasonings, and Spreads

Asparagus à la Sweet Lemon

PER SERVING: 128.4 CALORIES ~ 2.9 G PROTEIN ~ 6.2 G CARBOHYDRATE ~ 2.6 G FIBER ~ 11.3 G
TOTAL FAT ~ 1.7 G SATURATED FAT ~ 0.0 MG CHOLESTEROL ~ 293.7 MG SODIUM

Lemon is a great flavor to add to most dishes, and the nutmeg adds a surprising sweetness to the asparagus.

2 bunches asparagus (about 1 pound)

Juice of 1 medium lemon

3 tablespoons olive oil

½ teaspoon sea salt

¼ teaspoon black pepper

¼ teaspoon ground nutmeg

1 tablespoon ground cashews (for garnish)

Wash the asparagus, cut off the ends, and steam until the stems are cooked but still a little firm.

Mix together in a bowl lemon juice, oil, sea salt, pepper, and nutmeg. Arrange the asparagus on a serving dish and drizzle with the lemon juice mixture.

Garnish with ground cashews and serve immediately.

Serves 4.

Substitutions
You could try this recipe with green beans.

Healthy Tidbit
My parents have asparagus growing wild, and I love to graze on it (it's even tasty raw). Asparagus is the primary Ayurvedic root for strengthening female hormones. It also may promote fertility, increase lactation, and relieve menstrual pain. Asparagus can reduce phlegm and mucus, ease constipation, and is high in the powerful antioxidant glutathione. It has also been used in the treatment of heart failure, edema, rheumatism, and gout. To keep your asparagus fresh after purchase, stand it up in two inches of cold water in the refrigerator.

Nutritional Analysis per Serving			
Vitamin A	62.8 RE	Vitamin D	0.0 µg
Thiamin (B-1)	0.2 mg	Vitamin E	0.0 mg
Riboflavin (B-2)	0.2 mg	Calcium	30.1 mg
Niacin	1.1 mg	Iron	2.7 mg
Vitamin B-6	0.1 mg	Phosphorus	70.7 mg
Vitamin B-12	0.0 µg	Magnesium	22.7 mg
Folate (total)	53.2 µg	Zinc	0.7 mg
Vitamin C	10.7 mg	Potassium	257.6 mg

Baba Ghanoush

PER SERVING: 101.3 CALORIES ~ 3.2 G PROTEIN ~ 8.7 G CARBOHYDRATE ~ 3.8 G FIBER ~ 7.1 G
TOTAL FAT ~ 1.0 G SATURATED FAT ~ 0.0 MG CHOLESTEROL ~ 200.4 MG SODIUM

I used to go to this little Middle Eastern deli on my lunch break from
medical school, and it is there that I learned to love baba ghanoush. A
crowd pleaser, it is great for dipping and as a side to any meat dish.

1 large eggplant or 2 small eggplants

¼ cup plus 1 heaping tablespoon tahini (sesame seed butter, available
in most natural-food stores)

½–1 teaspoon salt

1–2 garlic cloves, minced

2 tablespoons fresh lemon juice

⅛ teaspoon ground cumin

¼ teaspoon black pepper

Paprika for garnish

Parsley for garnish

Preheat the oven to 350° F. Leaving the eggplant whole and unpeeled,
bake it on a baking sheet until soft, about 30 minutes. (For a smoother
baba ghanoush, remove the peel from the eggplant before blending.)
Allow to cool to room temperature.

Cut eggplant(s) open, remove as many seeds as you can, and cut the
remaining flesh into cubes. Blend all ingredients in blender until smooth.

Garnish with parsley and paprika, and serve with rice crackers, nonwheat bread, or dipping vegetables such as carrots and celery.

Serves 6.

Healthy Tidbit

Paprika, a relative of cayenne pepper, is ground from a sweet pepper in
the Solanaceae (nightshade) family. It is used often in Hungarian cooking
and has been used medicinally to prevent seasickness.

Nutritional Analysis per Serving			
Vitamin A	8.4 RE	Vitamin D	0.0 µg
Thiamin (B-1)	0.2 mg	Vitamin E	0.0 mg
Riboflavin (B-2)	0.1 mg	Calcium	28.7 mg
Niacin	1.3 mg	Iron	0.8 mg
Vitamin B-6	0.1 mg	Phosphorus	126.8 mg
Vitamin B-12	0.0 µg	Magnesium	25.7 mg
Folate (total)	33.5 µg	Zinc	0.8 mg
Vitamin C	5.1 mg	Potassium	280.1mg

Basil Pesto

PER SERVING: 330.6 CALORIES ~ 2.7 G PROTEIN ~ 4.1 G CARBOHYDRATE ~ 2.1 G FIBER ~ 35.1 G
TOTAL FAT ~ 4.3 G SATURATED FAT ~ 0.0 MG CHOLESTEROL ~ 146.8 MG SODIUM

This versatile pesto can be used on rice crackers, on nonwheat pasta, in egg dishes, in salads, or with anything else your taste buds can dream up. Spread it on a spelt pizza crust, or substitute it in any dish that calls for a tomato-based marinara sauce. You can double or triple the recipe and freeze the pesto in jars for future use.

4 cups fresh basil leaves, washed and patted dry

½ cup extra-virgin olive oil

3–4 cloves of garlic

¹/₃ cup pine nuts

¼ teaspoon salt

¼ teaspoon pepper (optional)

Process all ingredients in a food processor until smooth.
   Serves 4.

Substitutions

Pesto does not need to be made with basil; you can use cilantro, spinach, or parsley. You could even do a combination of two different herbs for variety. For example, use 2 cups basil with 2 cups spinach. You could also try using different nuts, such as walnuts or pecans.

Healthy Tidbit

Pine nuts give lubrication to the lungs and intestines. They are a great source of protein, can aid in coughs, and help to decrease constipation.

Nutritional Analysis per Serving			
Vitamin A	163.9 RE	Vitamin D	0.0 µg
Thiamin (B-1)	0.1 mg	Vitamin E	0.0 mg
Riboflavin (B-2)	0.1 mg	Calcium	71.6 mg
Niacin	0.9 mg	Iron	2.2 mg
Vitamin B-6	0.1 mg	Phosphorus	98.6 mg
Vitamin B-12	0.0 µg	Magnesium	63.7 mg
Folate (total)	31.1 µg	Zinc	1.1 mg
Vitamin C	8.4 mg	Potassium	273.6 mg

Cashew Cabbage

PER SERVING: 177.9 CALORIES ~ 6.6 G PROTEIN ~ 17.8 G CARBOHYDRATE ~ 4.5 G FIBER ~ 10.8 G
TOTAL FAT ~ 1.9 G SATURATED FAT ~ 0.0 MG CHOLESTEROL ~ 112.0 MG SODIUM

A version of this recipe has been in my family for generations. The cashews make the flavor very surprising and appealing.

1 small head of cabbage, chopped

2 stalks of celery

½ medium onion, chopped

Sea salt to taste

Pepper to taste

½ cup rice milk or soy milk (more or less, as needed)

1 cup ground cashews

Preheat oven to 350° F. Mix together cabbage, celery, onion, and seasonings, and place in a baking dish. Add rice milk or soy milk to cover; don't add too much. Bake until softened, about 50 minutes.

Top with ground cashews.

Serves 6.

Substitutions
Experiment with different seasonings. If you are able to tolerate a little dairy (see "Healthy Tidbit"), adding organic feta or goat cheese imparts a truly unique flavor.

Healthy Tidbit
Animal-based dairy products are very abundant in our culture and are consumed daily by most people. Because dairy is a common allergen, it is important to avoid or limit it in your cooking. Organic dairy products are better than regular dairy products because they lack the hormone, pesticide, and antibiotic residues that often are present in nonorganic animal products. Dairy allergies can cause chronic ear infections, chronic sinus infections, chronic skin rashes, postnasal drip, chronic cough or throat clearing, and many more minor symptoms.

Nutritional Analysis per Serving			
Vitamin A	21.4 RE	Vitamin D	0.0 µg
Thiamin (B-1)	0.2 mg	Vitamin E	0.2 mg
Riboflavin (B-2)	0.1 mg	Calcium	91.1 mg
Niacin	0.9 mg	Iron	2.3 mg
Vitamin B-6	0.2 mg	Phosphorus	163.9 mg
Vitamin B-12	0.0 µg	Magnesium	87.6 mg
Folate (total)	79.2 µg	Zinc	1.5 mg
Vitamin C	48.8 mg	Potassium	579.6 mg

Delicious Green Beans with Garlic

PER SERVING: 92.5 CALORIES ~ 2.8 G PROTEIN ~ 12.0 G CARBOHYDRATE ~ 4.0 G FIBER ~ 4.7 G TOTAL FAT ~ 0.7 G SATURATED FAT ~ 0.0 MG CHOLESTEROL ~ 342.6 MG SODIUM

I prepare this dish quite often. It is easy, quick, and always a crowd pleaser.

3 garlic cloves, minced or pressed

1 tablespoon plus 1 teaspoon olive oil

1 pound green beans, washed and trimmed

¼ cup filtered water

1 tablespoon plus 1 teaspoon tamari

2 teaspoons raw honey

In a large skillet, sauté the garlic in olive oil over medium heat for about 3 minutes.

Add the green beans, water, tamari, and honey, and cook over medium-low heat until beans are soft but still slightly crispy. If the water evaporates too quickly, keep adding water by the tablespoon—just enough to keep the beans steaming.

Serves 4.

Substitutions
I use this same recipe for asparagus and many other vegetables.

Healthy Tidbit
Fiber, provided in large quantities in lightly steamed, fresh vegetables, is essential to proper bowel function and should be increased in most people's diets. Adults need 25–30 grams daily (the average American's diet provides 10–12 grams). Low-fiber diets are associated with diverticulitis, cancers of the colon, and other gastrointestinal problems.

Nutritional Analysis per Serving			
Vitamin A	72.2 RE	Vitamin D	0.0 µg
Thiamin (B-1)	0.1 mg	Vitamin E	0.0 mg
Riboflavin (B-2)	0.1 mg	Calcium	47.5 mg
Niacin	1.1 mg	Iron	1.4 mg
Vitamin B-6	0.1 mg	Phosphorus	54.5 mg
Vitamin B-12	0.0 µg	Magnesium	31.4 mg
Folate (total)	36.9 µg	Zinc	0.3 mg
Vitamin C	16.4 mg	Potassium	260.6 mg

"French Fries"

PER SERVING: 181.4 CALORIES ~ 1.5 G PROTEIN ~ 43.2 G CARBOHYDRATE ~ 2.0 G FIBER ~ 0.3 G
TOTAL FAT ~ 0.1 G SATURATED FAT ~ 0.0 MG CHOLESTEROL ~ 15.9 MG SODIUM

I really missed fries, so I came up with this recipe when I learned that I could substitute a yucca root for potatoes. Now I can make them once in a blue moon and be satisfied for a long time before I crave fries again.

1 pound yucca root

Sea salt to taste

Pepper to taste

Steam or bake yucca roots until tender, about 40 minutes. When the yucca roots are nearly finished steaming, heat the oven to 375° F.

Allow yucca roots to cool enough so you can handle them. Cut off the outer waxy portion, and cut them into short sticks about ½ inch thick.

Place on a baking pan, add salt and pepper (and other seasonings, as desired), and bake until they reach the desired crispiness.

Serves 2–3.

Substitutions
You can do the same thing with sweet potatoes, which do not need to be steamed first. Also try taro root or Jerusalem artichokes (sunchokes).

Healthy Tidbit
A root poultice made from the yucca plant can treat skin sores and sprains. If decocted as a tea, it may ease arthritic pains.

Nutritional Analysis per Serving			
Vitamin A	2.3 RE	Vitamin D	0.0 µg
Thiamin (B-1)	0.1 mg	Vitamin E	0.0 mg
Riboflavin (B-2)	0.1 mg	Calcium	18.1 mg
Niacin	1.0 mg	Iron	0.3 mg
Vitamin B-6	0.1 mg	Phosphorus	30.6 mg
Vitamin B-12	0.0 µg	Magnesium	23.8 mg
Folate (total)	30.6 µg	Zinc	0.4 mg
Vitamin C	23.4 mg	Potassium	307.3 mg

Guacamole

PER SERVING: 145.0 CALORIES ~ 1.8 G PROTEIN ~ 8.2 G CARBOHYDRATE ~ 5.8 G FIBER ~ 13.1 G TOTAL FAT ~ 1.8 G SATURATED FAT ~ 0.0 MG CHOLESTEROL ~ 62.9 MG SODIUM

I have made this recipe since college, and it is always the talk of the party. It tastes so good with pretty much any dish. My favorite accompaniments are rice crackers, salads, rice and beans, poached organic eggs, or wheat-free, corn-free burrito wraps.

3 ripe avocados

2 garlic cloves, minced

2 tablespoons lemon juice

Sea salt to taste

Pepper to taste

2–3 tablespoons fresh cilantro, minced (optional)

1 teaspoon wheat-free tamari (optional; this will add salt, therefore reduce or exclude sea salt)

½–1 small onion, minced (optional)

Mash avocados with lemon juice. Add remaining ingredients and mix well. If you allow it to sit for ½ hour, the tastes really come together.

Serves 6.

Substitutions

Try the optional ingredients; they really make a flavorsome guacamole. Other vegetables to consider adding are chopped green pepper, chopped mild or medium pepper, green onions, chopped lettuce, puréed peas, or bean sprouts. They all add different elements. You can make your guacamole different every time. Adding more garlic will add more pungent flavor.

Healthy Tidbit

Cilantro, one of my favorite herbs, is a member of the carrot family. The seed, known as coriander, is sweet with a slight taste of orange peel. Cilantro is cooling and supports the spleen-pancreas, stomach, bladder, and lung meridians. It can regulate energy and has been used to aid digestion, and to relieve intestinal gas, pain, or bloating.

Nutritional Analysis per Serving			
Vitamin A	51.8 RE	Vitamin D	0.0 µg
Thiamin (B-1)	0.1 mg	Vitamin E	1.1 mg
Riboflavin (B-2)	0.1 mg	Calcium	13.4 mg
Niacin	1.7 mg	Iron	0.6 mg
Vitamin B-6	0.3 mg	Phosphorus	48.9 mg
Vitamin B-12	0.0 µg	Magnesium	25.5 mg
Folate (total)	76.3 µg	Zinc	0.6 mg
Vitamin C	10.1 mg	Potassium	442.4 mg

Nut 'n' Curry Hummus

PER SERVING: 356.0 CALORIES ~ 13.0 G PROTEIN ~ 31.9 G CARBOHYDRATE ~ 8.0 G FIBER ~ 21.9 G
TOTAL FAT ~ 2.4 G SATURATED FAT ~ 0.0 MG CHOLESTEROL ~ 300.9 MG SODIUM

This is another fabulous dipping sauce; it is the best-tasting hummus
recipe around. A colleague of mine, J.K. Monagle, N.D., inspired this
version. Using almond butter instead of peanut butter leaves nothing to
be desired. Thank you, J.K.

3 cups cooked garbanzo beans (2 cans)

¼ cup liquid from garbanzo beans

¹⁄₃ cup tahini (a sesame seed paste that can be purchased at most
health-food stores)

3 garlic cloves, minced or pressed

¼ cup plus 1 tablespoon fresh lemon juice

3 tablespoons filtered water

½–1 teaspoon sea salt, or to taste

½ cup almond butter

2 teaspoons curry powder

Paprika for garnish

Parsley for garnish

Blend all ingredients in blender until smooth.

Garnish with parsley and paprika, and serve with rice crackers, nonwheat bread, or fresh dipping vegetables such as carrots and celery.
Depending on the moisture content of your almond butter and tahini,
you may need to add a little extra water or lemon juice for blending.

Serves 6–8.

Substitutions

You can omit the almond butter and curry to make a plain hummus.
From the plain base, you can add different seasonings and vegetables, for
example, black olives, artichokes, spinach, or roasted red pepper.

Healthy Tidbit

Compared to many other
beans, garbanzo beans,
also known as chickpeas,
contain a fair amount of
vitamin C, which is an
important antioxidant.
Antioxidants function

Nutritional Analysis per Serving			
Vitamin A	4.3 RE	Vitamin D	0.0 µg
Thiamin (B-1)	0.3 mg	Vitamin E	0.0 mg
Riboflavin (B-2)	0.2 mg	Calcium	123.5 mg
Niacin	1.8 mg	Iron	4.0 mg
Vitamin B-6	0.2 mg	Phosphorus	359.9 mg
Vitamin B-12	0.0 µg	Magnesium	119.5 mg
Folate (total)	170.7 µg	Zinc	2.6 mg
Vitamin C	8.2 mg	Potassium	493.6 mg

within the body as free-radical scavengers, neutralizing many reactive oxygen species (ROS) before they can harm tissues. Free radicals occur normally in the body as a result of everyday metabolic reactions; in addition, certain dietary and lifestyle habits (e.g., smoking) tend to increase them. Increasing antioxidants in our diets is one way to protect ourselves from the free-radical damage that could eventually lead to chronic disease. According to an article by Ayako Makino appearing in the July 2003 issue of *Hypertension Journal,* oxidative stress caused by free radicals has been linked to high blood pressure and other cardiovascular diseases.

Lemon Vegetable Rice

PER SERVING: 304.9 CALORIES ~ 6.2 G PROTEIN ~ 50.4 G CARBOHYDRATE ~ 3.2 G FIBER ~ 9.7 G
TOTAL FAT ~ 1.6 G SATURATED FAT ~ 0.0 MG CHOLESTEROL ~ 397.2 MG SODIUM

For all those zucchinis we gardeners don't know what to do with in the fall, this is a terrific, light side dish that goes well with any dinner.

Juice of 2 medium lemons

2 tablespoons maple syrup

2½ cups of organic chicken broth

1½ cups of short-grain brown rice

½ teaspoon sea salt

1 cinnamon stick

5 whole cloves

2 tablespoons olive oil

1 teaspoon cumin seeds

1 small onion, thinly sliced

2 small zucchinis, sliced

1/3 cup roasted cashews, whole

2 tablespoons fresh sweet basil, chopped

Lemon wedges for garnish

Pour lemon juice, maple syrup, and chicken broth into a saucepan; add rice, sea salt, cinnamon stick, and cloves.

Cover, bring to a boil, and boil for 2 minutes. Reduce heat and simmer for 25–30 minutes or until all liquid has been absorbed.

In a large skillet, sauté cumin seeds in olive oil until they begin to pop. Add onion and cook for another 5 minutes over medium heat.

Add zucchini and cashews, and sauté until zucchini is tender.

Stir in the basil and the rice, heat for another minute or two, and serve garnished with lemon wedges.

Serves 6–8.

Substitutions

If you prefer a different type of nut, I would suggest pine nuts. If you don't have fresh basil, you can use any other fresh herb or leave that ingredient out.

Nutritional Analysis per Serving

Vitamin A	76.4 RE	Vitamin D	0.0 µg
Thiamin (B-1)	0.2 mg	Vitamin E	0.0 mg
Riboflavin (B-2)	0.1 mg	Calcium	52.5 mg
Niacin	2.5 mg	Iron	2.1 mg
Vitamin B-6	0.4 mg	Phosphorus	291.7 mg
Vitamin B-12	0.0 µg	Magnesium	104.6 mg
Folate (total)	36.0 µg	Zinc	1.9 mg
Vitamin C	19.5 mg	Potassium	507.6 mg

Healthy Tidbit

Lemons, like all citrus fruits, are a great source of vitamin C. They are also high in potassium and vitamin B-1, also known as thiamine. Lemons have less sugar and more acid, primarily citric acid, than any other citrus fruit. Lemon juice is antiseptic and astringent in addition to simulating saliva production, which aids in digestion. Lemon also promotes bile production, therefore supporting liver function. The essential oil of lemon is a stimulant and can help to purify water.

Mango Salsa

PER SERVING: 79.1 CALORIES ~ 0.9 G PROTEIN ~ 20.5 G CARBOHYDRATE ~ 2.3 G FIBER ~ 0.3 G
TOTAL FAT ~ 0.1 G SATURATED FAT ~ 0.0 MG CHOLESTEROL ~ 3.3 MG SODIUM

Of all the tomato dishes, salsa proved the hardest one for me to give up; therefore I had to come up with an alternative. You can use this version to replace salsa in any dish and to add a whole new dimension of flavor. It's perfect over a mildly seasoned white fish such as halibut. It also can complement guacamole or any Mexican dish.

3 ripe mangos, peeled and diced

1 red onion, minced

4 tablespoons finely chopped cilantro

Juice of ½ lemon

1–2 medium-spice peppers, such an Anaheim peppers (depending on your tolerance for spice)

Sea salt to taste

1 medium red bell pepper, minced (optional)

Combine all ingredients in a large bowl. Serve immediately with rice crackers, or store in the refrigerator. After it sits in the refrigerator for a little while, it tastes even better.

Serves 6–8.

Substitutions

You can experiment with adding anything you want, e.g., black beans, green bell peppers, avocado. You can even try adding other fruit such as kiwis or nectarines. If you cannot tolerate spice, leave out the hot peppers; it still tastes great.

Healthy Tidbit

Because mangos are cooling, they are great thirst quenchers. Mangos are high in vitamin-A precursors and vitamin C and are also a good source of potassium, which can aid in cardiovascular health. Mangos can be toning to all body types and constitutions.

Nutritional Analysis per Serving

Vitamin A	483.3 RE	Vitamin D	0.0 µg
Thiamin (B-1)	0.1 mg	Vitamin E	0.0 mg
Riboflavin (B-2)	0.1 mg	Calcium	15.7 mg
Niacin	0.7 mg	Iron	0.2 mg
Vitamin B-6	0.2 mg	Phosphorus	19.8 mg
Vitamin B-12	0.0 µg	Magnesium	13.1 mg
Folate (total)	20.2 µg	Zinc	0.1 mg
Vitamin C	42.4 mg	Potassium	216.7 mg

Mashed "Potatoes" (Mashed Jerusalem Artichokes)

PER SERVING: 80.4 CALORIES ~ 1.8 G PROTEIN ~ 13.5 G CARBOHYDRATE ~ 1.3 G FIBER ~ 2.4 G TOTAL FAT ~ 0.3 G SATURATED FAT ~ 0.0 MG CHOLESTEROL ~ 5.3 MG SODIUM

If you desire mashed potatoes at your Thanksgiving dinner, this is a great alternative.

1 pound Jerusalem artichokes, scrubbed

1 tablespoon olive oil

1 tablespoon fresh tarragon, chopped

2 tablespoons soy milk

Sea salt and pepper to taste

Preheat oven to 400° F.

Cut artichokes into wedges, toss with olive oil, and place in a baking pan. Bake for 35–40 minutes or until tender.

Remove from oven, mash well or pass through a food processor, and add remaining ingredients. Stir once more and serve warm.

Serves 6.

Substitutions

If you have a favorite mashed potato recipe, try it with Jerusalem artichokes. Just make sure to use a milk substitute, unless you can tolerate a little dairy. You can also steam cauliflower and use it in place of the Jerusalem artichokes. In place of tarragon, try oregano and/or thyme.

Healthy Tidbit

Jerusalem artichokes are a superior source of inulin, which is a compound beneficial for diabetics. They contain pro-vitamin A, B-complex vitamins, potassium, iron, calcium, and magnesium. They have been known to relieve asthmatic conditions, treat constipation, and nourish the lungs. It is best to purchase them during fall and winter, when their flavor peaks.

Nutritional Analysis per Serving			
Vitamin A	1.7 RE	Vitamin D	0.0 µg
Thiamin (B-1)	0.2 mg	Vitamin E	0.0 mg
Riboflavin (B-2)	0.0 mg	Calcium	13.3 mg
Niacin	1.0 mg	Iron	2.6 mg
Vitamin B-6	0.1 mg	Phosphorus	62.0 mg
Vitamin B-12	0.0 µg	Magnesium	14.4 mg
Folate (total)	10.7 µg	Zinc	0.1 mg
Vitamin C	3.0 mg	Potassium	335.1 mg

Milk Thistle Seasoning Salt

This blend is a tasty—and healthier—alternative to plain salt.

3 tablespoons milk thistle seeds (you can find these at a
health-food store)

3 tablespoons sea salt

Grind the milk thistle seeds in a coffee grinder until you have a fine powder. Mix with sea salt. Use as a replacement for regular salt.

Substitutions
Adding dried seaweed will afford even more nutrients. Just grind the seaweed in the coffee grinder and add the powder to the above mixture.

Healthy Tidbit
Milk thistle is specific in treating the liver, spleen, and kidneys. It is a very powerful protectant of the liver and is indicated for weak veins, blood stasis, and liver diseases. The liver is an important organ of detoxification.

Olive Oil–Butter Spread

PER SERVING: 107.7 CALORIES ~ 0.1 G PROTEIN ~ 0.0 G CARBOHYDRATE ~ 0.0 G FIBER ~ 12.2 G
TOTAL FAT ~ 5.5 G SATURATED FAT ~ 20.4 MG CHOLESTEROL ~ 54.6 MG SODIUM

I learned about this blend from my mentor, Dr. Dick Thom, who inspired this cookbook. Use it as a spread instead of plain organic butter or in cooking in place of plain organic olive oil.

1 pound organic butter, softened

1 cup extra-virgin olive oil

If necessary, heat the butter a little bit to facilitiate the blending of the ingredients. Mix well.

Store in refrigerator, and use sparingly as a spread.

Makes 48 servings of 1 tablespoon each.

Substitutions

Instead of olive oil you can use flaxseed oil or another high-omega-3 oil, but if you do, avoid heating it to high heat, such as for stir-frying vegetables. For stir-frying, just use olive oil or coconut oil.

Healthy Tidbit

Toxins such as heavy metals, pesticides, hormones, and antibiotics are stored in the body's fatty tissues. Therefore, it is important to purchase organic sources of foods that are high in fat. This is why only organic butter is allowed on the anti-inflammatory diet. Butter is superior to margarine, because the production of margarine usually involves hydrogenating plant oils to harden them for spreading. The body is physically unable to break down or digest the end results of this process (trans fatty acids). Hydrogenation also involves the use of heavy metals such as nickel, presenting the risk that they'll be present in the margarine. A few margarine products are now on the market that contain no dairy and are free of hydrogenated oils, such as Earth Balance margarine, which is also free of preservatives, genetically modified products, and artificial flavors. For more information on hydrogenated fats, please refer to Chapter 4.

Nutritional Analysis per Serving			
Vitamin A	47.3 RE	Vitamin D	0.1 µg
Thiamin (B-1)	0.0 mg	Vitamin E	0.0 mg
Riboflavin (B-2)	0.0 mg	Calcium	2.3 mg
Niacin	0.0 mg	Iron	0.0 mg
Vitamin B-6	0.0 mg	Phosphorus	2.3 mg
Vitamin B-12	0.0 µg	Magnesium	0.2 mg
Folate (total)	0.3 µg	Zinc	0.0 mg
Vitamin C	0.0 mg	Potassium	2.3 mg

"Peanut" Sauce

PER SERVING: 156.8 CALORIES ~ 2.7 G PROTEIN ~ 5.1 G CARBOHYDRATE ~ 1.9 G FIBER ~ 15.2 G TOTAL FAT ~ 10.4 G SATURATED FAT ~ 0.0 MG CHOLESTEROL ~ 88.8 MG SODIUM

Peanut sauce is a favorite accompaniment with Thai dishes such as salad rolls and saté skewers. Using almonds instead of peanuts loses none of the savory goodness. Red curry paste and fish sauce are available in Asian groceries or in the Asian aisle of most supermarkets.

5 ounces roasted, unsalted almonds	1 tablespoon honey
4 cups unsweetened coconut milk	3 tablespoons lemon juice
2 tablespoons red curry paste	3 teaspoons fish sauce

Blend the nuts in a coffee grinder, in small batches, until they are the consistency of fine meal.

In a large skillet, combine ½ of the coconut milk with the curry paste; cook over high heat until the mixture separates.

Then reduce heat, add the remaining ingredients plus the rest of the coconut milk, and heat over medium heat for 15–20 minutes, stirring occasionally.

Remove from heat and allow to sit for 20 minutes before serving. Serves 20.

Substitutions
You could try other roasted nuts instead of almonds. This recipe is easily cut in half to make a smaller amount of sauce. If this version is too spicy, reduce the amount of red curry paste.

Healthy Tidbit
Almonds and other nuts are excellent sources of protein. Almonds are also very high in calcium, B vitamins, iron, potassium, and phosphorus. They are one of the richest sources of vitamin E, which is a powerful anticancer antioxidant. Finally, substituting dietary calories with calories from almonds has a significant beneficial effect on lipid profiles, according to the results of a randomized feeding trial published in the June 1, 2003, issue of the *American Journal of Clinical Nutrition*.

Nutritional Analysis per Serving

Vitamin A	26.1 RE	Vitamin D	0.0 µg
Thiamin (B-1)	0.0 mg	Vitamin E	0.0 mg
Riboflavin (B-2)	0.1 mg	Calcium	27.4 mg
Niacin	0.7 mg	Iron	1.1 mg
Vitamin B-6	0.0 mg	Phosphorus	82.9 mg
Vitamin B-12	0.0 µg	Magnesium	39.8 mg
Folate (total)	10.8 µg	Zinc	0.6 mg
Vitamin C	5.4 mg	Potassium	185.1 mg

Poppy Seed Rice

PER SERVING: 150.6 CALORIES ~ 2.1 G PROTEIN ~ 24.3 G CARBOHYDRATE ~ 0.4 G FIBER ~ 4.8 G
TOTAL FAT ~ 0.7 G SATURATED FAT ~ 0.0 MG CHOLESTEROL ~ 0.3 MG SODIUM

This is a fun rice to serve when entertaining. I don't often use basmati rice because the glycemic index is much higher than brown rice, so I save this recipe for special occasions. You can create a very artistic meal using simple ingredients. Avoid this dish if you are diabetic.

1 cup basmati rice

2 cups filtered water

½ teaspoon sea salt (optional)

2 teaspoons fresh lemon juice

6 teaspoons olive oil or olive oil/butter mixture

1½ teaspoons poppy seeds

Lemon wedges for garnish

Wash and drain rice. Combine rice, water, sea salt, and lemon juice in a 2-quart saucepan over moderate heat. Bring to a boil.

In a small skillet, heat the oil over moderate heat; add the poppy seeds, and sauté until they become aromatic. Add seeds and oil to the boiling lemon juice, water, and rice; allow the water to fully boil for a few more seconds.

Reduce the heat to low, cover, and allow the rice to gently simmer without stirring or removing the lid for 15–20 minutes or until the rice is tender, dry, and fluffy. Turn off the heat and set aside for at least 5 minutes before serving.

Serves 6.

Substitutions
You can use brown rice, but it doesn't afford as much color contrast if you are looking for a creative, artistic presentation. It still tastes fabulous, however.

Healthy Tidbit
Poppy seeds are the dried seed of the opium poppy, *Papaver somniferum*, an herb native to Greece and the Middle East. Contrary to some myths, the seeds themselves have no narcotic

Nutritional Analysis per Serving			
Vitamin A	0.0 RE	Vitamin D	0.0 µg
Thiamin (B-1)	0.0 mg	Vitamin E	0.0 mg
Riboflavin (B-2)	0.0 mg	Calcium	10.3 mg
Niacin	0.0 mg	Iron	0.3 mg
Vitamin B-6	0.0 mg	Phosphorus	6.0 mg
Vitamin B-12	0.0 µg	Magnesium	2.4 mg
Folate (total)	0.6 µg	Zinc	0.1 mg
Vitamin C	0.8 mg	Potassium	7.0 mg

properties. Warming the seeds allows the flavors to come out. Poppy seeds have become popular in many dishes, from rice to salad dressings to sweet muffins. They are about half oil and thus can go rancid rapidly. Once you've opened a sealed container of them, store them in the refrigerator, tightly covered, and use them within a couple of months. To experiment with poppy seeds, try adding ¼ cup to a favorite muffin recipe.

Rosemary Squash

PER SERVING: 116.2 CALORIES ~ 1.4 G PROTEIN ~ 17.8 G CARBOHYDRATE ~ 2.6 G FIBER ~ 5.2 G
TOTAL FAT ~ 0.7 G SATURATED FAT ~ 0.0 MG CHOLESTEROL ~ 116.6 MG SODIUM

I first had this easy-to-prepare dish at a potluck supper when some of my
colleagues and I participated in a Native American sweat lodge. We
spent the day preparing for the sweat and getting the feast ready for
afterwards. After the sweat and thanking Mother Earth, everyone
enjoyed nourishing themselves on delicious food and great friendship.

2–3 small winter squash, such as acorn or spaghetti

2 medium sweet potatoes, unpeeled

3 tablespoons extra virgin olive oil

2 teaspoons rosemary

½ teaspoon sea salt or to taste

¼ teaspoon pepper or to taste

Cut the squash in half; spoon out the seeds and stringy flesh from the
center. Then cut into ³/₄-inch chunks, removing the shell.

Cut the sweet potatoes into ³/₄-inch chunks.

Combine sweet potatoes and squash in a large baking pan, drizzle
with olive oil, and add seasonings.

Cover and bake until squash chunks are tender but do not fall apart
when you fork them, about 40 minutes. Stir occasionally during the baking process.

Serves 8.

Substitutions
Try many different squash or pumpkin varieties for this dish, and omit
the sweet potatoes if you wish.

Healthy Tidbit
In recent years, rosemary has been the subject of research in the arena of
cancer prevention, Alzheimer's prevention and treatment, and heart disease treatment. Studies have shown that rosemary contains more than two
dozen antioxidants that may help prevent some of the most serious chronic

Nutritional Analysis per Serving			
Vitamin A	689.1 RE	Vitamin D	0.0 µg
Thiamin (B-1)	0.2 mg	Vitamin E	0.0 mg
Riboflavin (B-2)	0.0 mg	Calcium	46.3 mg
Niacin	0.9 mg	Iron	1.0 mg
Vitamin B-6	0.2 mg	Phosphorus	54.3 mg
Vitamin B-12	0.0 µg	Magnesium	42.9 mg
Folate (total)	22.1 µg	Zinc	0.2 mg
Vitamin C	12.7 mg	Potassium	485.5 mg

diseases. Because antioxidants are so important to cardiovascular health, rosemary has been looked at as a potentially cardio-protective herb. And in three separate studies on animals, rosemary has successfully inhibited the growth of cancer cells. More research on rosemary's anticancer effects will surely follow. One common use of rosemary is for its anti-inflammatory properties.

Salad Rolls

PER SERVING: 143.8 CALORIES ~ 11.7 G PROTEIN ~ 11.4 G CARBOHYDRATE ~ 2.2 G FIBER ~ 6.9 G
TOTAL FAT ~ 1.0 G SATURATED FAT ~ 0.0 MG CHOLESTEROL ~ 129.0 MG SODIUM

A favorite at Southeast Asian restaurants, such as those serving Thai or
Vietnamese cuisine, salad rolls are deceptively simple to make.

10 sheets of round rice paper (found in Asian section of the
grocery store)

Small package of rice noodles, cooked and rinsed

1 bunch of cilantro, minced or whole, with stems removed

½ pound of raw firm tofu, cut into long, thin strips

2 medium carrots, cut into long, thin strips

½ cucumber (cut lengthwise), cut into long, thin strips

Small amount of green leaf lettuce, shredded

Cut cilantro, tofu, carrots, cucumber, and lettuce as directed, and make a
pile of each for assembly.

Cook rice noodles according to package; rinse well with cold water
and set aside.

Fill a large saucepan ½ inch to 1 inch deep with filtered water and
heat over medium heat. Dip one sheet of rice paper into the water until it
softens (about 15–20 seconds). Remove from water, allow excess water
to drain off, and transfer to a cutting board.

One ingredient at a time, arrange a small amount of rice noodles,
cilantro, tofu, carrots, cucumbers, and lettuce on the bottom half of the
sheet of rice paper. Fold in the sides of the rice paper, and then roll
tightly into a large roll and set aside. Repeat with all ten sheets of rice
paper. You will learn how much of each ingredient fits into each roll by
experimenting. Cut each roll in half to expose the inside.

Serve immediately with wheat-free tamari or "Peanut" Sauce (see
recipe on page 72). Serves 10.

Substitutions

You can make these as
simple or complex as you
desire. Experiment with different vegetables, or even
add leftover fish. Adding
fresh mint instead of
cilantro also gives a crisp,
refreshing taste.

Nutritional Analysis per Serving			
Vitamin A	363.2 RE	Vitamin D	0.0 µg
Thiamin (B-1)	0.1 mg	Vitamin E	0.0 mg
Riboflavin (B-2)	0.1 mg	Calcium	473.6 mg
Niacin	0.4 mg	Iron	2.0 mg
Vitamin B-6	0.1 mg	Phosphorus	138.0 mg
Vitamin B-12	0.0 µg	Magnesium	43.2 mg
Folate (total)	24.2 µg	Zinc	1.1 mg
Vitamin C	1.8 mg	Potassium	227.8 mg

Healthy Tidbit

According to *Fast Food Nation,* by Eric Schlosser, in 1970 Americans spent $6 billion on fast food; in the year 2000, they spent over $110 billion, more than was spent on higher education, computers, computer software, or new cars. According to the Centers for Disease Control and Prevention (CDC), students can purchase name-brand fast foods, soda pop, candy bars, potato chips, and other high-fat, sugary snacks in 98.2 percent of American high schools. The fast food industry has become a quick fix in one sense, but a slow killer in another sense. Childhood obesity is on the rise; overweight in preschoolers is increasingly common. Long-term obesity can lead to hypertension, cardiovascular disease, diabetes, and other health complications.

Instead of bingeing on French fries and a shake, reeducate your palate to crave the healthful crunch of delicious homemade snacks such as these high-fiber salad rolls.

Scrumptious Green Beans

PER SERVING: 68.6 CALORIES ~ 1.5 G PROTEIN ~ 6.5 G CARBOHYDRATE ~ 2.7 G FIBER ~ 4.7 G
TOTAL FAT ~ 0.6 G SATURATED FAT ~ 0.0 MG CHOLESTEROL ~ 393.1 MG SODIUM

Simple green beans never tasted so good. This dish offers a great way to get some green vegetables into your family members' diets.

2 tablespoons olive oil

½ teaspoon black or yellow mustard seeds, available in the bulk herb
section of most health-food stores

½-inch cube of peeled ginger, sliced julienne thin

¼ cup water

1 pound green beans, washed and trimmed

½ teaspoon ground cumin

¼ teaspoon turmeric

1 teaspoon sea salt

2 tablespoons minced fresh cilantro

Juice of 1 lemon

Sauté mustard seeds and ginger in olive oil over moderate heat until mustard seeds begin to pop.

Add the beans and stir-fry over medium heat for about 5 minutes. Add the water, cover tightly, and simmer for 5 minutes.

Remove the lid when most of the water has evaporated. Add all remaining ingredients except lemon juice, and continue cooking until the beans are warm but still slightly crispy.

Add the lemon juice just before serving. Serve warm.

Serves 6.

Nutritional Analysis per Serving			
Vitamin A	48.5 RE	Vitamin D	0.0 µg
Thiamin (B-1)	0.1 mg	Vitamin E	0.0 mg
Riboflavin (B-2)	0.1 mg	Calcium	31.9 mg
Niacin	0.6 mg	Iron	0.9 mg
Vitamin B-6	0.1 mg	Phosphorus	30.3 mg
Vitamin B-12	0.0 µg	Magnesium	20.0 mg
Folate (total)	24.9 µg	Zinc	0.2 mg
Vitamin C	14.1 mg	Potassium	179.7 mg

Substitutions

If you have parsley on hand but not cilantro, try that instead. Use this recipe with many different vegetables, for example asparagus, sliced carrots, or root vegetables cut into long, thin strips. Remember, green beans also taste great steamed, without any seasonings. Try them prepared that way if you haven't already.

Healthy Tidbit

Green beans can act as a diuretic and may be helpful in diabetes. Fresh green beans are full of important nutrients such as pro-vitamin A, vitamin B-complex, calcium, and potassium. B vitamins offer support to the adrenals, which help to regulate blood sugar and blood pressure, produce some sex hormones, increase energy, and modulate the stress response.

Simple and Delectable Beets

PER SERVING: 26.8 CALORIES ~ 1.0 G PROTEIN ~ 6.0 G CARBOHYDRATE ~ 1.7 G FIBER ~ 0.1 G
TOTAL FAT ~ 0.0 G SATURATED FAT ~ 0.0 MG CHOLESTEROL ~ 48.0 MG SODIUM

Beets are so sweet that they really need no seasonings. But if you want to experiment with some new flavors, try this recipe.

3 beets, peeled and steamed until tender, but still slightly crunchy

1 teaspoon lemon juice

1 teaspoon honey (optional)

Sea salt and pepper to taste

Steam beets and set aside to cool slightly.

Mix lemon juice and honey together over low heat in a 2-quart saucepan until well blended.

Turn off heat, slice beets, and add them to the pan. Mix gently.

Add sea salt and pepper to taste, and serve immediately.

If you are omitting the honey, just slice the cooked beets, sprinkle with lemon juice, sea salt, and pepper, and serve.

Serves 4.

Substitutions

Use a dash of nutmeg or a bit of ginger instead of the honey to add flavor but no sugar.

Healthy Tidbit

Honey is my favorite sweetener. It is full of antioxidants and is mildly antiseptic. The Romans used it as a digestive healer, claiming it helped both diarrhea and constipation. Because it is easily absorbed, it satisfies the sweet tooth much better than other processed sugars. It is sweeter than cane sugar and it is unrefined. When replacing white sugar in a recipe with honey, use half as much honey as you would sugar (or even less). Because it has a higher water content than regular sugar, you can also cut the oil in half.

There, we have already made your recipe much healthier with one ingredient.

Nutritional Analysis per Serving			
Vitamin A	2.5 RE	Vitamin D	0.0 µg
Thiamin (B-1)	0.0 mg	Vitamin E	0.0 mg
Riboflavin (B-2)	0.0 mg	Calcium	9.9 mg
Niacin	0.2 mg	Iron	0.5 mg
Vitamin B-6	0.0 mg	Phosphorus	24.7 mg
Vitamin B-12	0.0 µg	Magnesium	14.2 mg
Folate (total)	67.2 µg	Zinc	0.2 mg
Vitamin C	3.6 mg	Potassium	201.4 mg

Steamed Vegetables

Steamed vegetables are the ideal accompaniment to many dinners. The combination of brown rice and steamed vegetables has become a popular Japanese-style quick food, called *bento*. Find a favorite anti-inflammatory sauce and serve it with brown rice and steamed vegetables. Here are some guidelines for steaming:

45 Minutes
Beets, carrots, turnips, winter squash, artichokes

25 Minutes
Sweet potatoes, broccoli stalks, peas, parsnips, celery

15 Minutes
Garlic, cabbage, sweet peppers, cauliflower, onions, green beans, asparagus

7 Minutes
Mushrooms, broccoli tips, zucchini, summer squash

Cut vegetables and place in steamer; cook for suggested length of time.
    Remove from heat, season, and serve warm.
Note: Using an electric steamer with a timer is best, because you can pay attention to your other cooking duties as your vegetables are steaming. If you do not have an electric steamer, use a metal steamer basket that fits into a saucepan or large pot; add an inch or so of water beneath it. This allows the vegetables to remain out of the water while cooking. If you do not have anything in which to steam vegetables, add a small amount of water to a saucepan or soup pot (enough water to cover the bottom), add the vegetables, and steam them over medium heat. You may have to add water as it evaporates, so be sure to watch closely to keep the vegetables from burning.

Healthy Tidbit
Insoluble fiber, contained in the cellulose of vegetables and the outer bran layer of whole grains, helps to increase stool bulk, stimulate normal gastrointestinal activity, and dilute colonic toxins. Insoluble fiber also helps to prevent the formation of diverticulosis. Soluble fibers are pectins, gums, mucilages, and some hemicelluloses. Sources include many fruits and vegetables, as well as oat bran, barley, and legumes. Soluble fibers aid in bacterial fermentation and act to bind bile salts, neutralizing them for excretion.

Stuffed Grape Leaves (Dolmades)

PER SERVING: 131.8 CALORIES ~ 2.5 G PROTEIN ~ 14.6 G CARBOHYDRATE ~ 2.6 G FIBER ~ 8.0 G
TOTAL FAT ~ 0.9 G SATURATED FAT ~ 0.0 MG CHOLESTEROL ~ 157.5 MG SODIUM

If you like lemony, tangy, and creative, this is your appetizer.

¾ cup cooked brown rice

4 ounces vine leaves such as grape leaves (these can be purchased in a
jar at an ethnic-food store)

1 tablespoon olive oil plus 1 tablespoon olive oil for sautéing

¼ cup minced onion

4 cloves garlic

2 tablespoons chopped mint leaves

¼ cup chopped fresh dill

$1/3$ cup raisins, chopped

$1/3$ cup pine nuts, chopped

1½ tablespoons chopped kalamata olives

¼ teaspoon sea salt

¼ teaspoon black pepper

¾ cup organic chicken broth

2 tablespoons lemon juice

Arrange grape leaves flat in bowl, cover with boiling water, and let sit
for 2 minutes. Drain, cover with cold water, let sit for 5 minutes, and
drain again.

Meanwhile, sauté onion and 1 minced garlic clove in 1 tablespoon
olive oil, stirring frequently, until soft, about 5 minutes.

Combine cooked rice, onion mixture, mint, dill, raisins, pine nuts,
olives, salt, and pepper in large bowl.

Preheat oven to 350° F. Place one leaf on cutting board, vein side
up, and cut off stem. Add a heaping spoonful of filling in the center.
Fold the sides of leaf over filling, then roll tightly from stem end to tip to
make a neat roll. If necessary, use a toothpick to keep each leaf neatly
rolled.

Set seam side down in a
wax paper–lined 9 x 13-inch
baking dish. Repeat with
remaining leaves and filling,
placing grape leaves cozily
together; make two layers if
necessary.

Nutritional Analysis per Serving			
Vitamin A	396.3 RE	Vitamin D	0.0 µg
Thiamin (B-1)	0.1 mg	Vitamin E	0.1 mg
Riboflavin (B-2)	0.1 mg	Calcium	65.9 mg
Niacin	0.9 mg	Iron	1.0 mg
Vitamin B-6	0.1 mg	Phosphorus	95.4 mg
Vitamin B-12	0.0 µg	Magnesium	39.5 mg
Folate (total)	16.7 µg	Zinc	0.6 mg
Vitamin C	4.5 mg	Potassium	177.1 mg

Cut 3 garlic cloves into large pieces and poke them here and there between the grape leaves. Pour chicken broth over grape leaves, then remaining olive oil and 1 teaspoon lemon juice. Bake 20–25 minutes, or until liquid is absorbed. Drizzle with remaining lemon juice and serve.

Serves 8.

Substitutions

I once met a woman who made the most wonderful stuffed grape leaves. When I asked her how she made them, she couldn't tell me the recipe because she said she makes them differently every time based on what she has in her kitchen. So be creative! You can add ½ pound of uncooked lamb to this recipe and increase the baking time to 35 minutes for a richer flavor.

Healthy Tidbit

Grape leaves are from a most versatile fruit. We eat grapes and we make wines and jams from them; we can even eat the leaves as a wrap for savory food ingredients. Grapes and grape leaves are a great source of vitamins A, B, and C.

Stuffed Mushrooms

PER SERVING: 317.7 CALORIES ~ 3.2 G PROTEIN ~ 5.8 G CARBOHYDRATE ~ 2.0 G FIBER ~ 32.8 G
TOTAL FAT ~ 7.0 G SATURATED FAT ~ 0.0 MG CHOLESTEROL ~ 5.9 MG SODIUM

Baked mushrooms, which can go with many meals, are a fun dish to make during the holidays. They are also good on the snack table at a party. You can experiment and serve three or four different kinds of stuffed mushrooms.

1 cup shredded, unsweetened coconut

25–30 small open-capped mushrooms, trimmed, with stems removed (simply pull them off)

1 cup olive oil

4 garlic cloves, minced

Juice of 2 lemons

Small amount of grated lemon zest (avoid the bitter white pith)

2 teaspoons grated gingerroot

¼ cup sunflower seeds, ground

Sea salt and pepper to taste

2 tablespoons chopped fresh cilantro leaves for garnish

Lemon wedges for garnish

Preheat oven to 400° F. Spread coconut on a baking sheet and bake until slightly browned.

Place mushrooms trimmed side up in a large roasting pan (use one that can go under the broiler).

Combine coconut with remaining ingredients in a large bowl and mix well. Spoon the mixture into the mushrooms evenly, cover loosely with foil, and bake 15–20 minutes or until mushrooms are tender. Broil at the last minute to brown the top. Serve garnished with lemon slices and cilantro leaves.

Serves 8.

Substitutions

You can use large mushrooms, such as portobellos, and make only 6–8 of them. For a variation on the stuffing, experiment with a combination of ground nuts, chopped spinach, olive oil,

Nutritional Analysis per Serving			
Vitamin A	0.5 RE	Vitamin D	1.1 µg
Thiamin (B-1)	0.2 mg	Vitamin E	0.0 mg
Riboflavin (B-2)	0.2 mg	Calcium	12.3 mg
Niacin	2.3 mg	Iron	1.0 mg
Vitamin B-6	0.1 mg	Phosphorus	94.6 mg
Vitamin B-12	0.0 µg	Magnesium	25.5 mg
Folate (total)	23.4 µg	Zinc	0.3 mg
Vitamin C	7.4 mg	Potassium	268.1 mg

and garlic. You may be surprised at how good vegetables and herbs can taste inside a mushroom.

Healthy Tidbit

Mushrooms are a powerful immune stimulant and immune modulator. They are great detoxifiers because they thrive upon what is decaying around them. They are said to absorb and safely eliminate toxins such as undesirable blood lipids, pathogens, and excess mucous in the respiratory system. The reishi and shiitake varieties have been studied for their anticancer effects. The reishi mushroom has been shown to reduce cancer-causing free radicals by 50 percent.

Sweet Potato "Fries"

PER SERVING: 93.8 CALORIES ~ 1.5 G PROTEIN ~ 19.6 G CARBOHYDRATE ~ 2.9 G FIBER ~ 1.2 G
TOTAL FAT ~ 0.2 G SATURATED FAT ~ 0.0 MG CHOLESTEROL ~ 51.0 MG SODIUM

This very simple recipe was given to me by Dawn Berry, L.Ac., an acupuncturist practicing in McMinnville, Oregon.

3 unpeeled sweet potatoes or yams, sliced into strips

1 teaspoon olive oil

Sea salt and pepper to taste

Dash of thyme

Dash of nutmeg

Preheat oven to 400° F. Toss olive oil, sweet potatoes, sea salt, and pepper in a large bowl.

Transfer to a baking pan, sprinkle with nutmeg and thyme, and bake for 30–35 minutes or until tender.

Serves 4.

Substitutions
Many different seasonings will work with sweet potatoes. Experiment with allspice, rosemary, or grated orange zest.

Healthy Tidbit
Fries from fast-food restaurants are cooked in oils at high temperatures, which means the oils have been converted to trans fatty acids and thus should be avoided. Furthermore, the familiar taste of fast-food fries is usually created by the addition of sugar, salt, and chemical flavorings. Sweet potato "fries" offer a much healthier alternative.

Nutritional Analysis per Serving			
Vitamin A	1,662.5 RE	Vitamin D	0.0 µg
Thiamin (B-1)	0.1 mg	Vitamin E	0.0 mg
Riboflavin (B-2)	0.1 mg	Calcium	27.8 mg
Niacin	0.5 mg	Iron	0.6 mg
Vitamin B-6	0.2 mg	Phosphorus	43.5 mg
Vitamin B-12	0.0 µg	Magnesium	23.2 mg
Folate (total)	9.7 µg	Zinc	0.3 mg
Vitamin C	1.8 mg	Potassium	295.7 mg

Vegetable Marinade for Grilling

PER SERVING: 323.9 CALORIES ~ 0.2 G PROTEIN ~ 1.2 G CARBOHYDRATE ~ 0.2 G FIBER ~ 36.1 G
TOTAL FAT ~ 5.0 G SATURATED FAT ~ 0.0 MG CHOLESTEROL ~ 389.0 MG SODIUM

Using this marinade causes the flavor of grilled vegetables to explode in your mouth. Serve them with a large salad and seasoned grilled fish.

1 cup olive oil

2 tablespoons red wine vinegar

5–7 cloves of garlic, finely chopped

½ teaspoon ground cayenne

½ teaspoon onion powder

½ teaspoon oregano

½ teaspoon black pepper

1 teaspoon sea salt

Whisk ingredients together with a fork until well blended. Paint vegetables with the marinade before and during the grilling process.

Serves 6.

Substitutions

For a lower-fat version, reduce the oil to ¼–½ cup and add ¼ cup of water. You can also use this recipe to marinate vegetables for a day before baking or steaming them. Chop the vegetables of your choice, place in a large Tupperware container, and pour marinade over the top. Periodically invert the container to consistently coat all the vegetables. Bake or broil the vegetables on a grate, which allows the oil to drain.

Healthy Tidbit

It is very important to meet our daily vitamin requirements through diet. In the U.S., vegetable intake has reduced significantly as incidence of noncommunicable disease has risen dramatically. Food is our source of fuel and energy, and vegetables hold the pure, vital, and essential nutrients we need to survive and thrive. Work on increasing your vegetable intake this week.

Nutritional Analysis per Serving

Vitamin A	7.1 RE	Vitamin D	0.0 µg
Thiamin (B-1)	0.0 mg	Vitamin E	0.0 mg
Riboflavin (B-2)	0.0 mg	Calcium	8.7 mg
Niacin	0.0 mg	Iron	0.4 mg
Vitamin B-6	0.0 mg	Phosphorus	5.4 mg
Vitamin B-12	0.0 µg	Magnesium	1.8 mg
Folate (total)	0.8 µg	Zinc	0.0 mg
Vitamin C	1.0 mg	Potassium	19.4 mg

Breads, Muffins, and Tortillas

Hannah's Rice-Flour Bread

PER SERVING: 533.9 CALORIES ~ 10.2 G PROTEIN ~ 96.7 G CARBOHYDRATE ~ 3.5 G FIBER ~ 12.1 G
TOTAL FAT ~ 6.0 G SATURATED FAT ~ 126.1 MG CHOLESTEROL ~ 740.1 MG SODIUM

Gluten-free bread has never tasted so good. Try this one; you won't be disappointed. This recipe is from Hannah Ashley, a massage therapist practicing in McMinnville, Oregon.

½ cup warm water

2 teaspoons plus ¼ cup honey

4 teaspoons dry yeast granules

2 cups rice flour

2 cups tapioca flour

4 teaspoons xanthan gum, available in health-food stores

1½ teaspoons sea salt

1¼ cups soy milk

4 tablespoons melted organic butter

1 teaspoon vinegar

3 organic eggs, gently beaten

In a small bowl, mix together water, 2 teaspoons honey, and yeast; set aside for 15 minutes.

In a large mixing bowl, combine dry ingredients.

Add wet ingredients to dry ingredients, and stir 20 times.

Add yeast mixture, and mix all with a mixer/beater. Note: Finished batter looks more like a thick cake batter than bread dough.

Divide batter into 2 equal amounts. Place in two 8 x 4 x 2½-inch, parchment paper–lined loaf pans. Smooth tops with a wet rubber spatula, and let rise in a warm place for approximately 1 hour.

Once dough has risen, preheat oven to 350° F. Bake loaves for 20–25 minutes. Serves 6.

Substitutions

You can experiment with different flours for this bread. You can also use any alternative milk in place of the soy milk. Coconut oil will easily replace the butter for those who can't tolerate any dairy.

Nutritional Analysis per Serving			
Vitamin A	95.1 RE	Vitamin D	0.5 µg
Thiamin (B-1)	0.2 mg	Vitamin E	0.0 mg
Riboflavin (B-2)	0.3 mg	Calcium	56.1 mg
Niacin	2.9 mg	Iron	2.0 mg
Vitamin B-6	0.3 mg	Phosphorus	180.7 mg
Vitamin B-12	0.3 µg	Magnesium	37.9 mg
Folate (total)	84.3 µg	Zinc	1.1 mg
Vitamin C	56.1 mg	Potassium	236.7 mg

Healthy Tidbit

An article published in 2005 in the journal *Bioscience, Biotechnology, and Biochemistry* indicates that bread containing resistant starch (6 grams or more of tapioca per 2 slices) is useful for prevention of lifestyle-related diseases such as type-II diabetes, and as a supplementary means of dietetic therapy. The resistant starch had an inhibitory effect on the postprandial (after eating) increase in blood glucose in male and female adults who had a fasting blood glucose level between 100 and 140 mg/dl.

Honey Millet Muffins

PER SERVING: 210.1 CALORIES ~ 5.3 G PROTEIN ~ 35.4 G CARBOHYDRATE ~ 2.7 G FIBER ~ 5.6 G
TOTAL FAT ~ 2.3 G SATURATED FAT ~ 26.5 MG CHOLESTEROL ~ 233.2 MG SODIUM

My daughter loves these little muffins, which can be served as a dessert because they taste so sweet.

1 organic egg

3 tablespoons organic butter, melted

½ cup milk substitute (e.g., soy milk) or water

½ cup honey

2 cups oat flour

1 teaspoon baking powder

½ teaspoon soda

½ teaspoon sea salt

1 cup millet, uncooked

½ teaspoon guar gum

Preheat oven to 375° F. Mix all wet ingredients together in a large bowl.

Still mixing, add the dry ingredients slowly. Add millet last, and stir through the mixture.

Spoon mixture into muffin tin (greased if you are not using paper liners), and bake for 17–20 minutes.

Makes 12 regular muffins.

Substitutions

This recipe contains enough guar gum to substitute for the gluten in wheat flour, so experiment with substituting different gluten-free flours. Oat happens to be my favorite because it tastes similar to whole wheat.

Healthy Tidbit

In the United States, millet is mostly used for bird feed, yet it would benefit us to include more of it in our diets. Millet is the preferred grain for treatment of blood sugar imbalances. Of all the cereal grains, it has the highest amount of protein and the highest iron content. It is also rich in phosphorus and the B vitamins.

Nutritional Analysis per Serving

Vitamin A	34.0 RE	Vitamin D	0.1 µg
Thiamin (B-1)	0.2 mg	Vitamin E	0.1 mg
Riboflavin (B-2)	0.1 mg	Calcium	41.1 mg
Niacin	1.1 mg	Iron	1.4 mg
Vitamin B-6	0.1 mg	Phosphorus	146.4 mg
Vitamin B-12	0.1 µg	Magnesium	46.6 mg
Folate (total)	23.5 µg	Zinc	1.0 mg
Vitamin C	0.1 mg	Potassium	126.5 mg

Spelt Bread

PER SERVING: 184.0 CALORIES ~ 4.7 G PROTEIN ~ 32.2 G CARBOHYDRATE ~ 4.5 G FIBER ~ 3.8 G TOTAL FAT ~ 2.4 G SATURATED FAT ~ 0.0 MG CHOLESTEROL ~ 349.7 MG SODIUM

Because spelt has gluten in it, this bread has no problem binding together without an additional binder. Use this as a substitute for wheat bread, but avoid eating it every day because of its gluten content and its allergic potential.

1 tablespoon active dry yeast

1¼ cups warm filtered water

2 tablespoons organic coconut oil, warmed to a liquid consistency

3 tablespoons raw honey or brown rice syrup

1½ teaspoon sea salt

3½–4½ cups spelt flour (final amount used will depend on humidity)

Mix ¼ cup warm water with yeast and let sit while preparing other ingredients.

In a large mixing bowl, mix 1 cup warm water, liquified coconut oil, honey, salt, and 1½ cups of flour. When the yeast is bubbly, add it to the mixing bowl. Beat generously for at least 60 seconds to develop the gluten. Add another cup of flour gradually while stirring the mixture to make a soft dough.

On a floured cutting board, knead the dough for 10 minutes while gradually adding more flour to form the dough into a round loaf. Add enough flour to keep the dough from sticking to the board but not so much that it falls apart. Avoid overworking the dough, which can lead to toughness.

When the loaf is finished, form it into a rectangle, place it in a greased bread pan, and set it in a warm place (85° F) to rise for 1 hour.

When the dough has risen slightly, bake at 350° F for 30 minutes. Remember, the spelt flour will cause the bread to rise less than it would with wheat flour; thus the loaf will be more dense than you are used to.

Makes one small loaf (approximately 10 servings).

Substitutions

You can add some baking powder to this recipe to help the bread rise a little more, but don't overdo it:

Nutritional Analysis per Serving			
Vitamin A	0.0 RE	Vitamin D	0.0 µg
Thiamin (B-1)	0.1 mg	Vitamin E	0.0 mg
Riboflavin (B-2)	0.1 mg	Calcium	1.4 mg
Niacin	1.8 mg	Iron	1.4 mg
Vitamin B-6	0.0 mg	Phosphorus	15.5 mg
Vitamin B-12	0.0 µg	Magnesium	1.3 mg
Folate (total)	27.8 µg	Zinc	0.1 mg
Vitamin C	0.0 mg	Potassium	186.1 mg

¼ to ½ teaspoon is plenty. If you want to shape the dough into buns, divide the loaf into 10 parts and shape them any way you desire before allowing them to rise.

You can try different combinations of flours, but remember, if the flour does not contain gluten, you also need to add a binder (see Substitutions Chart on page 226).

Healthy Tidbit

Although spelt is a relative of wheat and contains gluten, many wheat-intolerant people can tolerate it. As mentioned, because it contains a high amount of gluten, it should be rotated in the diet. Spelt's water solubility is different from wheat's and therefore it may be more readily assimilated into the body.

Spelt Tortillas

PER SERVING: 140.6 CALORIES ~ 3.4 G PROTEIN ~ 21.3 G CARBOHYDRATE ~ 3.4 G FIBER ~ 4.2 G
TOTAL FAT ~ 0.5 G SATURATED FAT ~ 0.0 MG CHOLESTEROL ~ 0.1 MG SODIUM

Tortillas can be served with many meals in place of bread or crackers.
This wheat-free, corn-free version is fun to make and tastes great.

2 cups spelt flour (option: 1 cup white spelt flour, 1 cup whole-grain spelt flour)

1 cup warm filtered water (slightly more or less depending on humidity level)

2 tablespoons olive oil

¼ cup spelt flour (for rolling out the dough)

Add water to spelt flour; knead the dough into a uniform mixture with
your hands. Form the mixture into 8 egg-sized balls; set aside for about
20 minutes.

On a generously floured surface, use a rolling pin to roll out 1 ball
into a circle. If the dough sticks to the rolling pin or the surface, add a
little more flour. If it falls apart, add a few drops of water.

Keep rolling the dough until you make a round, very thin tortilla.
(As you become more practiced, you will find it easier to make a round
shape; it is okay if your tortillas are not perfect the first time around.)

Heat a skillet over medium-high heat, and add ½ teaspoon olive oil.
Place the tortilla in the skillet, and heat it just enough to lightly brown
the bottom (about 60 seconds). When the tortilla is done on one side, it
will begin to puff up. Flip the tortilla and heat briefly on the other side
until lightly browned (about 60 more seconds).

Place directly into a napkin and fold the napkin over it to keep it
warm. Repeat with each dough ball. Serve immediately.

Makes 8 tortillas.

Healthy Tidbit

Making foods from scratch can prove beneficial to your health. When
you make tortillas at home, you are using only a few ingredients, all of
which you know are safe.
Next time you are in the
grocery store, pick up an
average package of tortillas and read the list of
ingredients. Tortillas are
simple and should remain
that way.

Nutritional Analysis per Serving			
Vitamin A	0.0 RE	Vitamin D	0.0 µg
Thiamin (B-1)	0.1 mg	Vitamin E	0.0 mg
Riboflavin (B-2)	0.0 mg	Calcium	0.0 mg
Niacin	1.0 mg	Iron	0.9 mg
Vitamin B-6	0.0 mg	Phosphorus	0.0 mg
Vitamin B-12	0.0 µg	Magnesium	0.0 mg
Folate (total)	0.0 µg	Zinc	0.0 mg
Vitamin C	0.0 mg	Potassium	127.9 mg

The All-Forgiving Banana Bread

PER SERVING: 368.5 CALORIES ~ 7.0 G PROTEIN ~ 42.3 G CARBOHYDRATE ~ 4.9 G FIBER ~ 20.8 G
TOTAL FAT ~ 6.7 G SATURATED FAT ~ 54.5 MG CHOLESTEROL ~ 232.2 MG SODIUM

I mean it when I say all-forgiving. You could do a lot to this recipe and still have it turn out great. Check out all the options in "Substitutions." Kids love this bread. Most people have no idea that it doesn't contain wheat. Compared to a regular banana bread recipe, it calls for only half the amount of butter/oil because it uses honey instead of sugar. It also contains half the amount of "sugar" of a regular banana bread.

¼ cup organic butter or vegan margarine (without hydrogenated oils), softened

¹/₈ cup organic coconut oil, warmed to a liquid consistency

½ cup honey

4 medium ripe bananas, puréed or thoroughly mashed with a fork

2 organic eggs

1 teaspoon baking soda

¼ teaspoon sea salt

1½ cup chopped walnuts

2 cups spelt flour

Preheat oven to 375° F.

Mix all wet ingredients together. You can use a blender to purée the bananas with the other wet ingredients. Gradually add the dry ingredients to the blender, and mix until smooth.

Pour into a 9 x 4 x 3-inch greased loaf pan or two small loaf pans. Bake for 15 minutes; reduce oven to 350° F and bake for another 40–45 minutes.

Makes one 9 x 4-inch loaf (approximately 10 slices).

Substitutions

As always, brown rice syrup is an acceptable substitute for honey. Plus, you can use pretty much any flour, or a combination of flours, and this recipe will turn out. Bananas add so much binder that they eliminate the need for the extra binder often called for when using a nonwheat

Nutritional Analysis per Serving			
Vitamin A	52.0 RE	Vitamin D	0.2 µg
Thiamin (B-1)	0.1 mg	Vitamin E	0.0 mg
Riboflavin (B-2)	0.1 mg	Calcium	27.7 mg
Niacin	1.3 mg	Iron	1.6 mg
Vitamin B-6	0.3 mg	Phosphorus	93.8 mg
Vitamin B-12	0.1 µg	Magnesium	42.8 mg
Folate (total)	32.3 µg	Zinc	0.8 mg
Vitamin C	4.4 mg	Potassium	362.8 mg

flour. My favorite is to use a combination of rice flour, garbanzo flour, and oat flour. Other options include rye flour and tapioca flour. As for the nuts, you can also experiment with pecans, cashews, pumpkin seeds, sunflower seeds, flaxseeds, coconut, or just about anything else you have in the cupboard. A small amount of raisins will add extra sweetness.

My favorite variation—always a crowd pleaser—is to use 1 cup coconut and 1 cup millet in place of the nuts; then pour the batter into muffin pans. Follow the baking directions in the recipe for honey millet muffins.

Healthy Tidbit
Ever since traveling to Africa, I have been curious about bananas. The bananas I ate there were unlike any I have eaten elsewhere, full of sweetness and moisture. I have been searching ever since for a banana that tastes that good. I was told there are 52 different species of bananas that grow on the African continent. Bananas are very high in potassium and therefore can help modulate blood pressure. They have a high sugar content, but are higher in minerals than any other soft fruit except strawberries (sadly, though, strawberries are often very heavily sprayed with chemicals).

Zucchini Bread

PER SERVING: 390.9 CALORIES ~ 6.7 G PROTEIN ~ 48.3 G CARBOHYDRATE ~ 2.3 G FIBER ~ 20.6 G
TOTAL FAT ~ 15.1 G SATURATED FAT ~ 63.5 MG CHOLESTEROL ~ 272.5 MG SODIUM

My mom made zucchini bread when I was little, and I love to eat it now
as much as I did then. You really can't taste the difference between the
old version and the healthy version.

¾ cup organic coconut oil, warmed to liquid consistency

3 organic eggs, beaten

2 cups grated zucchini

1 cup raw honey

1 teaspoon vanilla extract

3 cups oat flour

1 teaspoon baking soda

½ teaspoon sea salt

Preheat oven to 350° F.

Mix together all wet ingredients, including zucchini. Gradually add
dry ingredients, mixing thoroughly. Pour batter into a greased 9 x 4 x 3-
inch loaf pan.

Bake for 1 hour or until a knife inserted in the center comes out
clean. Makes one 9 x 4-inch loaf (approximately 10 slices).

Substitutions

You can try different combinations of flours with this recipe, but remember, if the flour does not contain gluten, you also need to add a binder.
Also experiment with adding seeds, chopped nuts, raisins, etc., for more
texture and varied flavor.

Healthy Tidbit

Zucchini are best if you eat them fresh and in season. They are great
from mid-summer through late fall. Look for locally grown varieties that
are small in size. They can
grow quite large, but the
larger they get the more
their flavor disappears.
When baked into cookies
and muffins, zucchini adds
moisture and important
nutrients.

Nutritional Analysis per Serving			
Vitamin A	36.3 RE	Vitamin D	0.2 µg
Thiamin (B-1)	0.2 mg	Vitamin E	0.0 mg
Riboflavin (B-2)	0.2 mg	Calcium	30.0 mg
Niacin	0.6 mg	Iron	1.7 mg
Vitamin B-6	0.1 mg	Phosphorus	174.2 mg
Vitamin B-12	0.2 µg	Magnesium	49.6 mg
Folate (total)	23.9 µg	Zinc	1.3 mg
Vitamin C	4.0 mg	Potassium	208.7 mg

Breakfasts

Five-Minute Breakfast

PER SERVING: 370.5 CALORIES ~ 11.0 G PROTEIN ~ 40.7 G CARBOHYDRATE ~ 5.2 G FIBER ~ 20.4 G
TOTAL FAT ~ 2.2 G SATURATED FAT ~ 0.0 MG CHOLESTEROL ~ 28.2 MG SODIUM

If you have leftover, cooked brown rice in your refrigerator, this is an easy meal, especially on those mornings when you think there's nothing in your kitchen for breakfast. I always make sure to have nuts, seeds, and raisins on hand for baked goods; therefore I always have the ingredients to make this simple breakfast.

1 cup leftover cooked brown rice	¼ cup sunflower seeds
¼ teaspoon cinnamon powder	½ cup rice milk or other alternative milk
⅛ cup raisins	¼ teaspoon carob powder (optional)
¼ cup chopped walnuts	½ teaspoon maple syrup (optional)

Combine all ingredients in a saucepan on the stove. Add milk to cover the rice for a cereal consistency. Warm over moderate heat to desired temperature and serve.

Serves 2.

Substitutions
Any seeds and nuts will do. Experiment with whatever is in your cabinet. Pumpkin spice or nutmeg would also be tasty. Or add fresh, cut fruit. You can always cook your rice fresh instead of using leftover rice, but the preparation time becomes longer than 5 minutes. Adding coconut milk instead of rice milk is a good way to add more fat to the diet and adds richer flavor.

Healthy Tidbit
Cinnamon-leaf oil can be used for its antiseptic, tonic, and warming properties. It is used to treat nausea and colds, and can be a powerful styptic, which means it can help halt bleeding. Research by Alam Khan and colleagues published in 2003 in the journal *Diabetes Care* suggests that cinnamon is helpful in regulating and stabilizing blood sugar.

Nutritional Analysis per Serving

Vitamin A	1.7 RE	Vitamin D	0.0 µg
Thiamin (B-1)	0.6 mg	Vitamin E	0.1 mg
Riboflavin (B-2)	0.1 mg	Calcium	64.0 mg
Niacin	2.7 mg	Iron	2.6 mg
Vitamin B-6	0.4 mg	Phosphorus	295.3 mg
Vitamin B-12	0.0 µg	Magnesium	142.8 mg
Folate (total)	66.6 µg	Zinc	2.2 mg
Vitamin C	0.8 mg	Potassium	378.3 mg

Broccoli and Olive Frittata

PER SERVING: 237.9 CALORIES ~ 15.2 G PROTEIN ~ 14.9 G CARBOHYDRATE ~ 2.3 G FIBER ~ 14.3 G
TOTAL FAT ~ 3.5 G SATURATED FAT ~ 317.3 MG CHOLESTEROL ~ 286.8 MG SODIUM

This is a great-tasting, crustless alternative to quiche.

1 medium yellow bell pepper

1 medium red bell pepper

2 broccoli crowns, cut into bite-size pieces

½ cup pitted ripe olives, halved

6 organic eggs, softly beaten

½ cup soy milk

2 tablespoons chopped fresh sweet basil or 1 teaspoon dried basil

1 teaspoon dried oregano

Sea salt and pepper to taste

¼ cup cashews, ground fine for garnish

Quarter and seed peppers, then broil them for 5–10 minutes or until lightly charred. Place in a closed brown paper bag, and let cool for 5 minutes. Peel and thinly slice. (If you don't mind the peel, leave it on and just slice the roasted peppers into thin slices.)

Reduce oven heat to 400° F.

Grease a 9-inch round pan. Place broccoli, peppers, and olives in the pan, making sure to arrange them evenly. Beat remaining ingredients together in a small bowl and pour over vegetables.

Bake for 35–40 minutes or until the center has set. Broil for the last two minutes to brown the top. Cool, slice into wedges, and serve warm or cold garnished with ground cashews (in place of Parmesan cheese).

Serves 4.

Substitutions

You can use this basic recipe for any type of frittata that you desire. Other ingredient ideas include basil, pine nuts, and pesto. You can add spinach to almost any frittata. Be creative.

Healthy Tidbit

Broccoli, as a member of the brassica family, supports liver function. It is

Nutritional Analysis per Serving			
Vitamin A	551.4 RE	Vitamin D	1.0 µg
Thiamin (B-1)	0.2 mg	Vitamin E	0.0 mg
Riboflavin (B-2)	0.5 mg	Calcium	120.1 mg
Niacin	1.5 mg	Iron	3.8 mg
Vitamin B-6	0.4 mg	Phosphorus	270.6 mg
Vitamin B-12	1.0 µg	Magnesium	68.9 mg
Folate (total)	115.9 µg	Zinc	1.9 mg
Vitamin C	208.6 mg	Potassium	609.7 mg

an important stimulator of the second phase of detoxification that occurs in the liver; therefore, try to include it in your diet often. It is also useful for eye complaints. A serving contains twice as much vitamin C as an orange and almost as much calcium as whole milk (and the calcium is better absorbed). It also contains selenium and vitamins pro-A and E. If you have a thyroid problem, consult a physician before eating broccoli raw.

Granola

PER SERVING: 317.9 CALORIES ~ 7.2 G PROTEIN ~ 24.3 G CARBOHYDRATE ~ 4.7 G FIBER ~ 23.4 G
TOTAL FAT ~ 10.3 G SATURATED FAT ~ 0.0 MG CHOLESTEROL ~ 3.3 MG SODIUM

This simple-to-make version of an old favorite allows you to avoid the additives and hydrogenated oils that are found in most commercially processed granola.

6 cups rolled oats	½ cup sesame seeds
1¼ cups unsweetened coconut	½ cup honey
1 cup chopped almonds	½ cup organic coconut oil
1 cup raw, shelled sunflower seeds	

Preheat oven to 325° F.

Mix dry ingredients together in a large bowl.

Combine honey and oil in a saucepan and heat to a liquid consistency. Pour over dry ingredients. Mix well. Flatten into a baking pan.

Bake for 15–20 minutes. Cool and store in an airtight container. Serve with milk substitute and/or fresh fruit.

Serves 14.

Substitutions

You can prepare this recipe with many different nuts and seeds and even dried fruit if you are not diabetic. For a change I sometimes add ½ cup of almond butter or tahini. You can also try brown rice syrup instead of honey.

Healthy Tidbit

The botanical name for oats is *Avena sativa*. One of my favorite medicinal uses for Avena is as an adrenal-supportive herb. It can help increase energy and tonify the adrenals while aiding anxiety or irritability. Because this herb supports the adrenals and energy production, it is an aid in balancing the endocrine system. I also use it for people who have difficulty sleeping related to overactive mind or anxiety. Eating oats has also been known to help decrease cholesterol.

Nutritional Analysis per Serving			
Vitamin A	0.7 RE	Vitamin D	0.0 μg
Thiamin (B-1)	0.4 mg	Vitamin E	0.0 mg
Riboflavin (B-2)	0.1 mg	Calcium	93.2 mg
Niacin	1.1 mg	Iron	2.6 mg
Vitamin B-6	0.2 mg	Phosphorus	0.3 mg
Vitamin B-12	0.0 μg	Magnesium	210.8 mg
Folate (total)	36.8 μg	Zinc	102.5 mg
Vitamin C	0.4 mg	Potassium	241.3 mg

Mexican Morning Eggs

PER SERVING: 303.7 CALORIES ~ 13.8 G PROTEIN ~ 29.4 G CARBOHYDRATE ~ 8.4 G FIBER ~ 16.1 G
TOTAL FAT ~ 3.4 G SATURATED FAT ~ 282.0 MG CHOLESTEROL ~ 734.0 MG SODIUM

I save this breakfast for when I have some leftover brown rice (and maybe some black beans) from the night before. It is simple and tastes delicious, and is filled with everything you need to begin your day. Adjust the amount of seasonings as necessary to satisfy your tastebuds.

4 organic eggs, cooked any way you like

1 cup leftover cooked brown rice

¾ cup black beans, home-cooked or from a can (rinse first to remove excess salt)

½ teaspoon cumin

½ teaspoon paprika

½ teaspoon chili powder

½ teaspoon sea salt

1 medium avocado, diced

Combine rice, beans, and seasonings in a skillet; cook over medium-low heat.

In a separate skillet, prepare eggs however you desire.

When eggs are finished and rice and beans are warm, serve them together on a plate. Add diced avocado on top.

Serves 3.

Substitutions
Experiment with other leftover grains, such as quinoa or amaranth. You can easily cut this recipe in half to accommodate fewer diners.

Healthy Tidbit
Many people are concerned about the cholesterol content of eggs. In fact, however, eggs have in them an anticholesterol agent that protects our bodies from their cholesterol content. I believe that eggs can be good dietary cholesterol regulators. Organic eggs especially are good cholesterol regulators, because the chickens' diet contains fewer toxins. If the chickens were fed flaxseeds, eggs would be an even better regulator. Remember from earlier in the book that eggs need to be cooked slowly. Otherwise, enjoy!

Nutritional Analysis per Serving			
Vitamin A	198.5 RE	Vitamin D	0.9 µg
Thiamin (B-1)	0.2 mg	Vitamin E	0.0 mg
Riboflavin (B-2)	0.4 mg	Calcium	84.6 mg
Niacin	2.2 mg	Iron	2.9 mg
Vitamin B-6	0.4 mg	Phosphorus	214.3 mg
Vitamin B-12	0.9 µg	Magnesium	53.7 mg
Folate (total)	85.1 µg	Zinc	1.6 mg
Vitamin C	6.7 mg	Potassium	607.8 mg

Protein Power Breakfast

PER SERVING: 343.6 CALORIES ~ 10.1 G PROTEIN ~ 30.3 G CARBOHYDRATE ~ 8.8 G FIBER ~ 23.1 G
TOTAL FAT ~ 2.7 G SATURATED FAT ~ 0.0 MG CHOLESTEROL ~ 7.0 MG SODIUM

This quick and easy breakfast is filled with many nutrients, including essential fatty acids and protein.

1 tablespoon flaxseeds	1 teaspoon honey
2 tablespoons sesame seeds	½ medium banana, sliced
2 tablespoons sunflower seeds	

Grind all seeds together in your coffee grinder (which by now must be going through an identity crisis).

Place seeds in a cereal bowl. Add honey and a small amount of hot water or hot milk substitute. Mix together and top with sliced bananas.

Sprinkle a little more honey or maple syrup on top and enjoy.

Serves 1.

Substitutions

According to taste, you can use different combinations of seeds. I also like to add ground coconut. For a cold version of the breakfast, substitute cold milk in place of the hot water.

Healthy Tidbit

Flaxseeds are an excellent source of omega-3 fatty acids because of their alpha-linolenic acid component. Essential fatty acids are called "essential" because our body cannot make them; therefore we must obtain them through diet. Our body is quite dependent upon the balance of important fats in the diet. Omega-3 and omega-6 fatty acids must be in balance to promote eicosanoid formation. Eicosanoids are precursors to important hormone-like compounds that help to regulate the body's endocrine system, inflammatory processes, and overall metabolism. The typical American diet currently provides up to thirty times more omega-6 fatty acids than omega-3 fatty acids, which can promote an imbalance in the inflammatory processes and increase susceptibility to disease. This is why it is vitally important to consume a variety of foods and to make sure you get plenty of omega-3 fatty acids. See Chapter 4 for more on this topic.

Nutritional Analysis per Serving

Vitamin A	5.8 RE	Vitamin D	0.0 µg
Thiamin (B-1)	0.8 mg	Vitamin E	0.0 mg
Riboflavin (B-2)	0.2 mg	Calcium	230.4 mg
Niacin	2.4 mg	Iron	4.7 mg
Vitamin B-6	0.6 mg	Phosphorus	330.4 mg
Vitamin B-12	0.0 µg	Magnesium	190.0 mg
Folate (total)	80.7 µg	Zinc	2.9 mg
Vitamin C	5.5 mg	Potassium	520.7 mg

Quickest Oatmeal You'll Ever Eat

PER SERVING: 297.7 CALORIES ~ 8.2 G PROTEIN ~ 68.4 G CARBOHYDRATE ~ 6.2 G FIBER ~ 4.2 G
TOTAL FAT ~ 0.7 G SATURATED FAT ~ 0.0 MG CHOLESTEROL ~ 196.7 MG SODIUM

This breakfast takes fewer than three minutes to prepare. For an on-the-go version, use a glass bowl with a tightly sealed lid, place all the ingredients in it, and add it to the contents of your briefcase or backpack. If you've used boiling water, when you get to work or school, your cereal will be cool enough to eat.

1 cup nut-and-fruit muesli (natural with no additives)

½–1 cup hot or boiling water

½ teaspoon maple syrup (optional; the fruit in the cereal adds sweetness)

Stir all ingredients together in a cereal bowl. Let sit for at least 1 minute before eating.

Serves 1.

Substitutions

Another quick idea for hot cereal is to begin with 1 cup plain oatmeal, add a few frozen berries and a little honey, and pour boiling water over the mix. The water will melt the berries, making the oatmeal ready to eat in about 60 seconds. Adding ground flaxseeds to your oatmeal increases the fiber, protein, and essential fatty acids.

Healthy Tidbit

When Mom said to eat breakfast every morning, she was right. Research presented at the American Heart Association's 43rd annual conference, in March 2003, showed that breakfast-eaters are far less likely to be obese or have diabetes or heart disease. Eating a whole-grain cereal each day was associated with a 15 percent reduction in risk for insulin resistance syndrome, a precursor to diabetes and weight gain.

Nutritional Analysis per Serving			
Vitamin A	0.0 RE	Vitamin D	0.0 µg
Thiamin (B-1)	0.8 mg	Vitamin E	0.0 mg
Riboflavin (B-2)	0.9 mg	Calcium	2.2 mg
Niacin	10.3 mg	Iron	7.5 mg
Vitamin B-6	1.0 mg	Phosphorus	206.6 mg
Vitamin B-12	3.1 µg	Magnesium	66.8 mg
Folate (total)	206.6 µg	Zinc	3.2 mg
Vitamin C	0.0 mg	Potassium	419.9 mg

Tofu Scramble

PER SERVING: 114.4 CALORIES ~ 7.5 G PROTEIN ~ 10.1 G CARBOHYDRATE ~ 2.6 G FIBER ~ 5.7 G
TOTAL FAT ~ 1.0 G SATURATED FAT ~ 0.0 MG CHOLESTEROL ~ 224.1 MG SODIUM

Tofu is a good alternative to eggs for breakfast. This recipe has been adapted from *The Complete Food Allergy Cookbook*, by Marilyn Gioannini, M.D.

1 pound firm tofu

2 tablespoons spelt flour (or any type of nonwheat flour)

1 tablespoon olive oil, for sautéing

4–5 cups chopped mixed vegetables (for example, zucchini, yellow squash, carrots, onions, and garlic)

1 teaspoon onion powder

1 teaspoon paprika

2 teaspoons garlic powder

½ teaspoon sea salt

½ teaspoon turmeric

1 teaspoon curry powder

Black pepper to taste

Dash cayenne if tolerated

½ cup filtered water

Drain tofu of extra moisture and cut into slabs.

Mix spices and flour together in a small bowl.

If using garlic and onions, sauté them together in a large skillet over medium heat until they are soft. Add other vegetables, and continue sautéing until they are partially cooked.

Add tofu by crumbling it into pieces to resemble scrambled eggs. Add spice/flour mixture and water.

Sauté a little longer until vegetables are cooked to your liking. (Make sure to cook flour long enough to eliminate the taste of raw starch—about 2 minutes). Serve immediately.

Serves 6.

Substitutions

Use any vegetables you want; this is a good way to clean out your crisper drawer of small amounts of leftover raw veggies. For a time-saving measure, quadruple the seasoning and flour mixture, and store the extra in a small jar for the next few times you make the recipe.

Nutritional Analysis per Serving			
Vitamin A	597.8 RE	Vitamin D	0.0 µg
Thiamin (B-1)	0.1 mg	Vitamin E	0.0 mg
Riboflavin (B-2)	0.1 mg	Calcium	172.0 mg
Niacin	0.5 mg	Iron	1.7 mg
Vitamin B-6	0.2 mg	Phosphorus	120.9 mg
Vitamin B-12	0.0 µg	Magnesium	39.1 mg
Folate (total)	30.3 µg	Zinc	0.8 mg
Vitamin C	6.8 mg	Potassium	305.5 mg

Healthy Tidbit

The soybean is a magical bean. Even five thousand years ago, Chinese texts referred to the soybean as one of the most important crops. Soy is an inexpensive source of vegetarian protein. It is rich in isoflavones (a plant estrogen) and therefore is often suggested to menopausal women for prevention of osteoporosis and alleviation of some menopausal complaints.

I need to caution against soy and its possible allergenicity. Some people can react to soy, so it should be experimented with. To determine whether you react to soy, leave it out of your diet for four weeks, and then reintroduce it (see the section in Chapter 3 on food allergies and intolerances for a discussion of how to test yourself for food sensitivities). Because of its many uses, the soybean is often genetically modified or heavily processed, increasing its potential for allergenicity. Buying organic soy products is one way to lessen potential reactions.

Dr. Fisel's Tofu Scramble

PER SERVING: 140.5 CALORIES ~ 12.1 G PROTEIN ~ 7.0 G CARBOHYDRATE ~ 2.9 G FIBER ~ 8.4 G
TOTAL FAT ~ 1.5 G SATURATED FAT ~ 0.0 MG CHOLESTEROL ~ 277.7 MG SODIUM

I have gained inspiration for many vegetarian dishes from my good
friend Matt Fisel, N.D.

1 tablespoon olive oil	1 tablespoon nutritional yeast powder
½ onion, chopped	2 teaspoons kelp powder (optional)
1 clove garlic, chopped	1 teaspoon cumin powder
5 mushrooms, sliced	¼ teaspoon cayenne powder (omit if you
1 cup chopped broccoli	can't tolerate spice)
1 1-pound package organic, firm tofu, crumbled	1 tablespoon wheat-free tamari
	Pepper to taste
2 teaspoons Herbes de Provence	Salt to taste

In a large skillet, heat the oil; add the onions, garlic, mushrooms, and
broccoli. Sauté on medium-high heat until the onions are translucent.

Add crumbled tofu to pan. Add all of the remaining ingredients and
sauté until moisture has evaporated and vegetables are tender, about 10
minutes.

Serves 4.

Substitutions
You can use any vegetables for this scramble, even leftover vegetables.

Healthy Tidbit
Tofu, made from soybean curd, is an inexpensive, high-quality source of
protein. Soy is a good source of iron, phosphorus, potassium, sodium,
and calcium. It also provides B vitamins, choline, and vitamin E.

Nutritional Analysis per Serving			
Vitamin A	40.2 RE	Vitamin D	0.4 µg
Thiamin (B-1)	0.4 mg	Vitamin E	0.0 mg
Riboflavin (B-2)	0.3 mg	Calcium	253.7 mg
Niacin	2.0 mg	Iron	2.6 mg
Vitamin B-6	0.2 mg	Phosphorus	217.1 mg
Vitamin B-12	0.0 µg	Magnesium	56.7 mg
Folate (total)	120.8 µg	Zinc	1.4 mg
Vitamin C	21.5 mg	Potassium	412.5 mg

Wheat-Free Pancakes

PER SERVING: 208.1 CALORIES ~ 4.2 G PROTEIN ~ 27.0 G CARBOHYDRATE ~ 2.7 G FIBER ~ 9.4 G
TOTAL FAT ~ 1.0 G SATURATED FAT ~ 0.0 MG CHOLESTEROL ~ 500.95 MG SODIUM

This recipe comes from a colleague who has exceptional talent in the cooking arts, Erika Siegel, N.D., L.Ac.

½ cup walnuts, ground in food processor to a fine powder

¾ cup spelt flour

¾ cup rice flour

1 teaspoon cream of tartar

1 teaspoon baking soda

¾ teaspoon sea salt

1 ⅓ cup water

1 tablespoon olive oil

Optional—sprinkle fresh berries, chopped apple, or chopped nuts into batter.

Combine ground walnuts, flours, salt, cream of tartar, baking soda, and salt in a medium-sized mixing bowl, blending well.

Whisk 1 cup of water into dry ingredients, then gradually add the rest of the water to reach desired consistency. Add more water if the batter is still too thick. Stir in any optional ingredients until just combined.

Brush or spray a large skillet or griddle with small amount of oil. Heat skillet or griddle over medium heat. Drop batter onto hot cooking surface using a large spoon. Cook the pancake until bubbles form on top; flip. Cook on the second side until lightly browned.

Serves 6.

Substitutions

You can try other nuts (e.g., pecans) and other types of flour. If you replace the spelt flour with a nongluten flour, you may need to add ¼–½ teaspoon guar gum or a blended banana.

Healthy Tidbit

Many people have wheat allergies or sensitivities. Symptoms can be as severe as celiac disease, in which no gluten is tolerated at all and results in gastrointestinal damage, or as minor as

Nutritional Analysis per Serving			
Vitamin A	0.4 RE	Vitamin D	0.0 µg
Thiamin (B-1)	0.1 mg	Vitamin E	0.0 mg
Riboflavin (B-2)	0.0 mg	Calcium	12.0 mg
Niacin	1.1 mg	Iron	0.8 mg
Vitamin B-6	0.1 mg	Phosphorus	54.0 mg
Vitamin B-12	0.0 µg	Magnesium	22.7 mg
Folate (total)	10.6 µg	Zinc	0.5 mg
Vitamin C	0.1 mg	Potassium	198.5 mg

postnasal drip, cough, or phlegm. It is well documented that many neurological conditions are related to gluten intolerance as a result of nutrient deficiency due to malabsorption. Another newer theory is that gluten proteins may cause direct immunological reactions within brain, nerve, and muscle tissue, independent of the gastrointestinal system. If you suffer from any neurological condition, it is worth a 4-week trial of gluten-avoidance.

Easy Pancakes

PER SERVING: 322.7 CALORIES ~ 18.4 G PROTEIN ~ 15.9 G CARBOHYDRATE ~ 2.7 G FIBER ~ 21.6 G
TOTAL FAT ~ 4.4 G SATURATED FAT ~ 317.3 MG CHOLESTEROL ~ 120.7 MG SODIUM

These pancakes, which have a delicious nutty flavor, offer a high amount of fiber and can be made with virtually no flour.

3 tablespoons raw sunflower seeds, ground fine

3 tablespoons raw pumpkin seeds, ground fine

3 organic eggs

¼ cup nongluten oat flour (any nonwheat or nongluten flour will do)

¼ cup rice milk

¼ cup blueberries (optional)

Combine all ingredients in a medium-sized bowl and mix well until clumps have dissolved.

Heat a lightly oiled skillet or griddle pan over medium heat.

Pour batter into 3-inch diameter circles in the pan. When pancakes begin to bubble, flip and cook on the other side for a short amount of time until lightly browned on both sides.

Serves 2.

Substitutions

You may add berries or other fruit to this recipe. If the fruit is frozen, the batter has a tendency to clump around it; the pancakes still turn out fine. Ben Unterseher, a massage therapist in McMinnville, Oregon, converted this recipe into an amazing flat bread that is similar to pita bread. He added 1 tablespoon fresh ground rosemary, 1 clove minced garlic, ½ cup garbanzo flour, ½ cup soy flour (omit the oat flour above), 2 eggs instead of 3, 1 tablespoon sea salt, and ½ cup filtered water. Pour batter in 6-inch diameter circles instead of 3-inch and cook similarly.

Healthy Tidbit

With the rise in incidence of celiac disease (gluten intolerance), a demand has developed for people to find alternatives to high-gluten foods. Gluten reactions can include diarrhea, abdominal pain, bloating,

Nutritional Analysis per Serving			
Vitamin A	148.8 RE	Vitamin D	1.0 µg
Thiamin (B-1)	0.5 mg	Vitamin E	0.0 mg
Riboflavin (B-2)	0.5 mg	Calcium	72.8 mg
Niacin	1.1 mg	Iron	4.9 mg
Vitamin B-6	0.3 mg	Phosphorus	459.3 mg
Vitamin B-12	1.0 µg	Magnesium	149.0 mg
Folate (total)	80.6 µg	Zinc	3.0 mg
Vitamin C	0.4 mg	Potassium	378.0 mg

flatulence, pallor, weakness, fatigue, and behavioral changes such as irritability and depression, weight loss, delayed growth in children, missed menstrual periods, bone and joint pain, seizures, muscle cramps, and others. Complete gluten avoidance can improve and elimate most of these symptoms in celiac disease sufferers.

Breakfast Eggnog

PER SERVING: 303.3 CALORIES ~ 19.6 G PROTEIN ~ 20.4 G CARBOHYDRATE ~ 0.0 G FIBER ~ 12.9 G
TOTAL FAT ~ 3.6 G SATURATED FAT ~ 423.0 MG CHOLESTEROL ~ 226.1 MG SODIUM

This is a very easy breakfast to whip together for yourself or your children and offers a good source of complete protein in the morning.

2 organic eggs

1 cup rice milk, chilled

1 tablespoon vanilla extract

Dash cinnamon

Dash nutmeg

Combine all ingredients in a large cup or bowl, and mix well until mixture looks uniform.

Strain mixture through small strainer into a serving glass and serve. Serves 1.

Substitutions

Soy milk or another alternate milk can be used in place of rice milk.

Healthy Tidbit

Many individuals are nervous when they see raw eggs in a recipe due to the chance of getting salmonella poisoning. This is a valid concern, but the risk of contracting salmonella from eggs is actually significantly low. The U.S. Department of Agriculture has indicated that salmonella incidence fell by 66 percent from 1998 to 2003. In the healthy individual, salmonella poisoning is a self-limiting disease that is quickly recovered from. Symptoms of salmonella poisoning include diarrhea, abdominal pain, nausea, vomiting, fever, and chills. It mostly strikes the elderly, infants, and those with compromised immune systems such as cancer or HIV sufferers.

Nutritional Analysis per Serving			
Vitamin A	191.0 RE	Vitamin D	1.3 µg
Thiamin (B-1)	0.2 mg	Vitamin E	0.0 mg
Riboflavin (B-2)	0.6 mg	Calcium	94.4 mg
Niacin	0.5 mg	Iron	3.0 mg
Vitamin B-6	0.2 mg	Phosphorus	291.8 mg
Vitamin B-12	1.3 µg	Magnesium	53.5 mg
Folate (total)	73.0 µg	Zinc	2.0 mg
Vitamin C	0.0 mg	Potassium	422.6 mg

Breakfast Smoothie

PER SERVING: 601.2 CALORIES ~ 41.1 G PROTEIN ~ 79.1 G CARBOHYDRATE ~ 14.4 G FIBER ~ 15.7 G TOTAL FAT ~ 1.9 G SATURATED FAT ~ 0.0 MG CHOLESTEROL ~ 1073.9 MG SODIUM

This fast, simple breakfast can sustain your blood sugar until midmorning or lunch. Once you get the hang of it, you can make a smoothie in less than five minutes, transfer it to a jar or mug, and be out the door, almost as quickly as if you'd skipped breakfast. Make the time; it is worth it.

2 tablespoons soy protein powder

1 cup organic frozen berries (blueberries, strawberries, raspberries, blackberries, cherries)

2 cups soy milk (use water if you prefer, or half water and half milk)

Place all ingredients in blender and blend to desired thickness and consistency. Serves 1–2.

Substitutions

You can use a rice-based protein powder, or, instead of protein powder, you can use ½ block or more of silken tofu. Also, you can use any milk substitute (e.g., rice milk, almond milk).

You may add the following ingredients based on your tastebuds and your dietary needs. If you do so, you may need to use more liquid:

½–1 frozen banana, cut into chunks

2 tablespoons freshly ground flaxseeds (highly recommended)

1–3 teaspoons flaxseed oil or other omega-3 fatty acid oil

1 teaspoon vanilla extract

1–2 teaspoons acidophilus or fructo-oligosaccharides

Healthy Tidbit

Eating enough protein with each meal is an important way to regulate blood sugar levels. Consistently healthy levels of blood sugar lead to consistent energy levels and fewer mood swings. Furthermore, having high blood sugar for an extended period of time can lead to diabetes, high blood-lipid levels, and high cholesterol levels.

Nutritional Analysis per Serving			
Vitamin A	387.9 RE	Vitamin D	0.0 µg
Thiamin (B-1)	0.8 mg	Vitamin E	0.5 mg
Riboflavin (B-2)	0.3 mg	Calcium	736.6 mg
Niacin	8.1 mg	Iron	8.7 mg
Vitamin B-6	0.3 mg	Phosphorus	767.7 mg
Vitamin B-12	0.0 µg	Magnesium	222.8 mg
Folate (total)	229.9 µg	Zinc	4.4 mg
Vitamin C	27.1 mg	Potassium	1,315.4 mg

Teas and Other Beverages

Herbal "Juice"

This tea is an excellent replacement for fruit juice. Every child loves juice, and here is a substitute without all the added sugars. And the hibiscus makes it a very pretty red. Even if you sweeten the tea a little bit, it will still be healthier than store-bought juice. Your kids won't know the difference! All ingredients should be available in the bulk section of a well-stocked natural-foods store.

½ cup dried crataegus (hawthorn) leaves
½ cup dried crataegus (hawthorn) berries
½ cup rose hips
¼ cup dried hibiscus flowers

½ cup dried peppermint leaves
Zest of 1 medium lemon
Honey to taste (optional)

Mix all ingredients together and store in an airtight container for use as needed. For each serving, use 1 tablespoon of tea mixture and 10 fluid ounces (1¼ cup) of filtered water. For a gallon of tea (approximately 12 servings), use a gallon of filtered water and 12 tablespoons (¾ cup) of tea mixture.

In a tea kettle (for small quantities) or a large pot, bring water to a boil. Remove from heat, add dried herbs and lemon zest, and allow to steep for 10–15 minutes.

Filter into a large container through a very fine strainer or 2–3 thicknesses of cheesecloth. When tea is still warm, add honey to taste and store in refrigerator. Serve chilled (or, if you desire, warm).

Yield: 2¼ cup dried tea mix, or approximately 36 servings.

Substitutions
Explore the dried-herb section of the bulk-foods department for many different teas to blend together to suit your tastes and those of your children. Be creative and adventurous.

Healthy Tidbit
According to a 2003 study by Cornell University, children who drank more than 12 ounces of sweetened drinks daily gained significantly more weight than children who drank less than 6 ounces. The sweetened drinks were classified as soda, fruit punch, lemonade, or similar drinks.

Hawthorn, which tastes great in teas and tinctures, is a wonderful healing herb. It supports circulation and cardiac function, including regulation of blood pressure, by dilating blood vessels. Besides being used for both high and low blood pressure, it has been used to treat heart weakness, arteriosclerosis, and irregular heartbeat. It also offers calming support of the heart chakra, which can lighten the mood.

The remainder of this section offers recipes for various caffeine-free teas that taste delicious and soothing served warm, or refreshing and invigorating served cool.

Instructions for brewing tea appear at the end.

Chai

PER SERVING: 61.5 CALORIES ~ 3.5 G PROTEIN ~ 9.2 G CARBOHYDRATE ~ 0.1 G FIBER ~ 1.6 G
TOTAL FAT ~ 0.3 G SATURATED FAT ~ 0.0 MG CHOLESTEROL ~ 43.0 MG SODIUM

3 cups rice milk

3 cups water

1 cinnamon stick, 2 inches long

8 whole black peppercorns

2 whole cloves

4 cardamom seeds

½ teaspoon whole cumin seeds

¼ teaspoon ground allspice

1/8 teaspoon ground nutmeg

Serves 6.

Nutritional Analysis per Serving			
Vitamin A	0.3 RE	Vitamin D	0.0 µg
Thiamin (B-1)	0.1 mg	Vitamin E	0.0 mg
Riboflavin (B-2)	0.1 mg	Calcium	23.3 mg
Niacin	0.2 mg	Iron	0.7 mg
Vitamin B-6	0.0 mg	Phosphorus	51.2 mg
Vitamin B-12	0.0 µg	Magnesium	21.1 mg
Folate (total)	13.1 µg	Zinc	0.5 mg
Vitamin C	0.1 mg	Potassium	140.5 mg

Calming Tea

2 parts chamomile flowers

1 part passionflower

1 part hypericum (St. John's wort)

1 part lavender flowers

The Stress Reliever

2 parts oatstraw
2 parts lindenflower
1 part passionflower
1 part lemon balm

Adrenal Support Tea (for energy)

1 part Siberian ginseng
1 part gotu kola
1 part ginkgo biloba
1 part licorice

Simple Mood Tea (to lift the spirits)

1 part passionflower
1 part lemon balm
1 part hypericum (St. John's wort)

Cleansing Tea (No steeping necessary)

Juice of ½ lemon
1 tablespoon pure maple syrup
8–10 ounces filtered water, cold or hot
¼ teaspoon cayenne (decrease if you can't tolerate the spiciness)

Detoxification Tea

1 part burdock root
1 part dandelion root
2 parts licorice root

Tea to Relax the Nerves

1 part hibiscus flowers
1 part basil
1 part catnip
1 part lemon balm
2 parts peppermint

Easy Digestion Tea

2 parts peppermint
1 part fennel
1 part anise seed
½ part gingerroot

Immune Booster Tea

2 parts elderberry
2 parts echinacea
1 part licorice
1 part hyssop
1 part thyme
2 parts peppermint

Sleepy Tea

2 parts chamomile
2 parts skullcap
1 part passionflower
1 part valerian (optional)

Instructions

There are two different ways to make teas: infusion and decoction. Most teas are infusions, created when herbs are placed in very hot water and left to steep for about 15 minutes. A decoction is used when roots are involved. For a decoction, the roots need to be boiled for a time before steeping to bring out their medicinal quality.

For an Infusion
Follow instructions for Herbal "Juice" on page 117.

For a Decoction
Use 1 tablespoon tea blend per 10 fluid ounces (1¼ cup) of filtered water. In a saucepan or kettle, place the root only (not other ingredients) in water and bring to a boil.

Cover, reduce heat to medium, and allow the water to simmer for 15–25 minutes.

Remove from the burner and allow the tea to steep another 10 minutes, covered. If there are other herbs to infuse with this tea, add them at this time.

Filter through a very fine strainer or 2–3 thicknesses of cheesecloth.

Substitution Ideas
These tea blends are not set in stone; they're just suggestions. I usually make teas based on what I have in my herb cupboard. If I am missing some ingredients, I use others in their place. Remember, you are the creative mastermind in your own kitchen. If you want to add lemon zest, hibiscus flowers, honey, or other ingredients to your teas to make them more palatable, feel free.

These teas are not medical treatments and are not meant to take the place of medical treatment. If you have a serious condition, consult with your naturopathic physician.

Almond Milk

PER SERVING: 105.3 CALORIES ~ 4.0 G PROTEIN ~ 3.6 G CARBOHYDRATE ~ 1.9 G FIBER ~ 9.2 G
TOTAL FAT ~ 0.7 G SATURATED FAT ~ 0.0 MG CHOLESTEROL ~ 5.1 MG SODIUM

Almond milk, which is very simple to make, is superior to cow's milk because of its reduced allergen potential and its significant content of plant-based essential fatty acids. When you're short on time, you can buy almond milk in the health-food section of grocery stores or at any natural-foods store.

1 cup raw, whole almonds

3 cups filtered water (more or less, depending on desired taste and consistency)

Soak the almonds overnight in a small amount of filtered water.

Drain off the water. Rub each almond between your fingers to remove the brown skin. Blend the skinned almonds with a small amount of fresh filtered water at a high speed until they reach a smooth consistency.

After blending, add water to reach desired taste and thickness. Then, strain the milk through a fine strainer or two layers of cheesecloth. You may add sweetener, but it is usually not needed if you use fresh almonds.

Serves 4.

Substitutions

If you want to make the recipe a little faster and simpler, use slivered almonds, which do not have any peel to rub off after soaking.

You can make milk from many different kinds of nuts. Not all nuts need to be soaked overnight to remove the peel. Always start by blending the nuts with a small amount of water, then adding more water to desired taste and consistency.

Healthy Tidbit

Almonds contain a considerable amount of highly absorbable calcium. One-fourth cup of almonds provides 92 mg of calcium. The calcium in cow's milk is not absorbed optimally due to milk's allergenicity; therefore, almond milk is a better alternative as a calcium source. It is also much

Nutritional Analysis per Serving			
Vitamin A	0.2 RE	Vitamin D	0.0 µg
Thiamin (B-1)	0.0 mg	Vitamin E	0.0 mg
Riboflavin (B-2)	0.1 mg	Calcium	39.2 mg
Niacin	0.7 mg	Iron	0.7 mg
Vitamin B-6	0.0 mg	Phosphorus	87.0 mg
Vitamin B-12	0.0 µg	Magnesium	49.8 mg
Folate (total)	5.4 µg	Zinc	0.6 mg
Vitamin C	0.0 mg	Potassium	124.5 mg

less inflammatory. According to the principles of Ayurvedic medicine, almonds help to mildly alkalinize the system and strengthen bones, nerves, and the reproductive system. Almond milk also offers protein, essential fatty acids, and important nutrients such as B vitamins, iron, potassium, vitamin E, and phosphorus.

Sesame Milk

PER SERVING: 121.5 CALORIES ~ 3.2 G PROTEIN ~ 9.5 G CARBOHYDRATE ~ 2.6 G FIBER ~ 8.9 G
TOTAL FAT ~ 1.3 G SATURATED FAT ~ 0.0 MG CHOLESTEROL ~ 2.6 MG SODIUM

This milk is jam-packed with important nutrients and protein. It's a great way to get some nutrition into your children. I like to mix equal parts sesame milk and rice milk for a scrumptious drink on the rocks.

1 cup sesame seeds

3½ cups filtered water

1 tablespoon honey

2 teaspoons carob powder

Grind the seeds in a coffee grinder and combine with remaining ingredients in a large container. Shake thoroughly, and let sit for 15 minutes.

Shake again and strain through 2 thicknesses of cheesecloth or a very fine strainer. Chill in the refrigerator or serve over ice. Keep refrigerated.

Serves 4.

Substitutions
Experiment with other seeds or seed mixtures.

Healthy Tidbit
Sesame seeds are rich in fiber, essential fatty acids, potassium, iron, phosphorus, and vitamins A, E, B-1, B-3, B-6, and folic acid. Make sure to buy unhulled sesame seeds to ensure nutrient conservation as many of the nutrients are removed during the hulling process. Products such as tahini often use hulled seeds; it is better to purchase tahini made from seeds that have been hulled mechanically as opposed to chemically. Chemically hulled sesame seeds have often been exposed to lye, which denatures their protein and nutrients and sacrifices taste. Sesame seeds contain over 35 percent protein, which is more than any nut contains.

Nutritional Analysis per Serving			
Vitamin A	0.2 RE	Vitamin D	0.0 µg
Thiamin (B-1)	0.1 mg	Vitamin E	0.0 mg
Riboflavin (B-2)	0.0 mg	Calcium	179.5 mg
Niacin	0.8 mg	Iron	2.7 mg
Vitamin B-6	0.1 mg	Phosphorus	114.3 mg
Vitamin B-12	0.0 µg	Magnesium	63.9 mg
Folate (total)	17.9 µg	Zinc	1.4 mg
Vitamin C	0.0 mg	Potassium	95.8 mg

Entrées

Baked Tofu

PER SERVING: 280.0 CALORIES ~ 17.7 G PROTEIN ~ 17.1 G CARBOHYDRATE ~ 0.9 G FIBER ~ 17.9 G
TOTAL FAT ~ 2.1 G SATURATED FAT ~ 0.0 MG CHOLESTEROL ~ 1,353.9 MG SODIUM

One of my favorite dishes because it is so versatile, baked tofu can be stir-fried with veggies and served over rice (using the extra marinade in a sauce), eaten in a sandwich with sprouts, or added to a salad of mixed greens with a savory dressing.

1 pound extra-firm tofu

2 tablespoons sesame oil

4 tablespoons wheat-free tamari

2 tablespoons honey

3 garlic cloves, minced

1½ teaspoons grated fresh ginger

Drain tofu of excess water by placing it between two towels and putting something heavy on top. I use a medical textbook, because it is heavy enough to squeeze out any extra water.

While the tofu is drying, mix together in a sealable container sesame oil, tamari, honey, garlic, and ginger. (If you want more marinade, just increase the liquids proportionally.)

Slice the tofu into chunks or slabs, and marinate for at least 1 hour (1 full day is better). Turn tofu periodically by inverting the container.

Bake at 375° F on a baking sheet for 10–15 minutes or until browned. Flip and bake for 10–15 more minutes until browned. Broiling for an extra 3 minutes produces a crispier tofu.

Serves 3.

Substitutions

The marinade is still yummy even without the garlic and ginger, so if you're feeling a little lazy, just skip them. You may also try the marinade with fish or chicken; it works well with just about anything.

Healthy Tidbit

An article by Brunilda Nazario, M.D., appearing in *webMD Medical News* on April 28, 2003, stated that sesame oil may decrease blood pressure. There are two great reasons

Nutritional Analysis per Serving

Vitamin A	1.5 RE	Vitamin D	0.0 µg
Thiamin (B-1)	0.1 mg	Vitamin E	0.0 mg
Riboflavin (B-2)	0.1 mg	Calcium	275.8 mg
Niacin	1.4 mg	Iron	0.1 mg
Vitamin B-6	0.2 mg	Phosphorus	242.3 mg
Vitamin B-12	0.0 µg	Magnesium	91.2 mg
Folate (total)	30.5 µg	Zinc	1.8 mg
Vitamin C	1.8 mg	Potassium	273.9 mg

to include sesame oil in your diet. First, it is rich in mono- and polyun-saturated acids (PUFAs), which are the good kinds of fat that lower blood cholesterol levels. Second, it is low in saturated fats, which are the kind that you should limit in your diet. Sesame oil also contains two very powerful antioxidants: sesamol and sesamin.

Barbequed Kafta

PER SERVING: 336.8 CALORIES ~ 26.1 G PROTEIN ~ 2.4 G CARBOHYDRATE ~ 0.6 G FIBER ~ 24.0 G
TOTAL FAT ~ 9.4 G SATURATED FAT ~ 114.9 MG CHOLESTEROL ~ 120.2 MG SODIUM

Easy-to-make kafta is always pleasing. Impress guests with a Mediterranean meal of kafta, hummus with rice crackers (instead of pita bread), brown rice, and cucumber salad.

1 pound ground lamb

1 pound ground turkey

1 onion, grated or finely minced

²/₃ cup finely chopped parsley

¼–½ teaspoon cayenne

½ teaspoon allspice

¼–½ teaspoon black pepper

Metal or wooden skewers

Mix all ingredients together well.

Take a small amount of the mixture and press firmly around the length of a skewer. Repeat this process until all of the mixture is gone.

Bake or grill the skewers until browned. Serve over rice.

Serves 6.

Substitutions
You could use all lamb, but adding turkey reduces the richness of the lamb.

Healthy Tidbit
Did you know that parsley can freshen your breath? Maybe that is why it is found in so many dishes containing garlic. Parsley is rich in vitamins and minerals, is an excellent antioxidant, and improves digestion. If you are planning an herb garden, plant your parsley next to your roses; it improves their health and fragrance.

Nutritional Analysis per Serving			
Vitamin A	39.9 RE	Vitamin D	0.0 µg
Thiamin (B-1)	0.1 mg	Vitamin E	0.0 mg
Riboflavin (B-2)	0.3 mg	Calcium	36.8 mg
Niacin	7.3 mg	Iron	2.6 mg
Vitamin B-6	0.4 mg	Phosphorus	246.0 mg
Vitamin B-12	2.0 µg	Magnesium	35.9 mg
Folate (total)	32.8 µg	Zinc	4.1 mg
Vitamin C	10.3 mg	Potassium	412.1 mg

Blackened Salmon

PER SERVING: 201.2 CALORIES ~ 27.1 G PROTEIN ~ 4.1 G CARBOHYDRATE ~ 1.5 G FIBER ~ 9.0 G
TOTAL FAT ~ 1.7 G SATURATED FAT ~ 43.1 MG CHOLESTEROL ~ 883.7 MG SODIUM

Blackened salmon is always a hit. Vary the level of spice depending on who will be joining you for dinner.

1–2 fillets wild salmon (approximately 12 ounces total)

For the seasoning
1 tablespoon garlic powder
1 tablespoon dried parsley flakes
1 tablespoon dried basil

2 teaspoons thyme
1–2 teaspoons cayenne pepper
1 teaspoon sea salt
¼ teaspoon ground black pepper
1 tablespoon olive oil (for cooking)

Mix seasonings together and spread onto a flat plate. Invert the salmon into the seasoning, then flip over, making sure to coat all areas.

Heat olive oil in a skillet over medium-high heat. Before the oil begins to smoke, place salmon flesh-side down in the pan. Turn the salmon after about 3 minutes. Continue cooking until flesh is still a little rare in the middle when tested with a small knife, about 2–3 more minutes. Serve over fresh spring greens with a simple dressing such as vinegar and oil.

Serves 3.

Substitutions

Use this basic blackening season for fish, chicken, or turkey.

Healthy Tidbit

Cayenne has many uses. Because of its capsaicin constituent, it can be used topically to treat pain from arthritis, shingles, neuralgia, and pleurisy. Initially it may exacerbate pain, so use it with caution or with supervision. Cayenne has also been used to treat colds, fevers, varicose veins, and asthma.

Nutritional Analysis per Serving			
Vitamin A	54.1 RE	Vitamin D	18.0 µg
Thiamin (B-1)	0.1 mg	Vitamin E	1.1 mg
Riboflavin (B-2)	0.1 mg	Calcium	106.2 mg
Niacin	17.7 mg	Iron	3.0 mg
Vitamin B-6	0.9 mg	Phosphorus	844.5 mg
Vitamin B-12	3.7 µg	Magnesium	46.9 mg
Folate (total)	11.5 µg	Zinc	0.9 mg
Vitamin C	2.7 mg	Potassium	541.0 mg

Breaded Red Snapper with Mango Salsa

PER SERVING: 435.2 CALORIES ~ 31.8 G PROTEIN ~ 36.2 G CARBOHYDRATE ~ 6.4 G FIBER ~ 20.6 G
TOTAL FAT ~ 2.9 G SATURATED FAT ~ 93.9 MG CHOLESTEROL ~ 120.3 MG SODIUM

Who said you had to give up breading on your fish? This very simple
recipe is made even simpler if you prepare the mango salsa ahead of time
or the day before. Your guests will compare this meal favorably with any
they could get in a restaurant.

16 ounces red snapper fillets (about 4 small fillets)

¼ cup sesame seeds, ground fine

¼ cup sunflower seeds, ground fine

¼ cup almonds, ground fine

1 organic egg

1 tablespoon olive oil

Sea salt to taste

Mango Salsa (recipe on page 68)

In a medium-sized bowl, beat the egg with a small amount of water until
mixed thoroughly.

Pour ground sesame seeds onto a flat plate, ground sunflower seeds
onto another plate, and ground almonds onto a third plate.

Dip one fillet through the egg mixture, and coat with ground sesame
seeds by pressing it into the seeds, turning the fillet over to repeat on the
other side. You may have to use your hands to cover all areas of the fillet
with ground seeds. Set this fillet aside.

Repeat with the next fillet, this time coating it in ground almonds.
Repeat with a third fillet, coating it with sunflower seeds. After you are
finished, you should have at least one fillet with each type of coating.

Brush olive oil over a baking sheet. Arrange coated fillets on the
baking sheet and bake at 375° F for 10–15 minutes, until fish is flaky
but still moist when tested carefully with a small knife.

You can also cook the fish in a nonstick skillet with a very small
amount of oil over medium
heat. Cook the fillets on
both sides until flaky but
still moist, turning once
after about three minutes.

Serve with mango salsa
spooned over the top.

Serves 4.

Nutritional Analysis per Serving			
Vitamin A	787.3 RE	Vitamin D	0.2 µg
Thiamin (B-1)	0.6 mg	Vitamin E	0.0 mg
Riboflavin (B-2)	0.4 mg	Calcium	171.2 mg
Niacin	6.1 mg	Iron	3.6 mg
Vitamin B-6	0.5 mg	Phosphorus	357.3 mg
Vitamin B-12	0.2 µg	Magnesium	106.9 mg
Folate (total)	67.7 µg	Zinc	1.7 mg
Vitamin C	63.7 mg	Potassium	812.4 mg

Substitutions

Try other ground seeds (e.g., pumpkin). If you have just one type of seed, use it to coat all the fillets. You can use any white fish, for example sole, tilapia, cod, halibut. If you are unable to tolerate eggs, simply drag the fillets through warmed coconut oil before coating them with the seed mixture.

Healthy Tidbit

Part of the pleasure of indulging in wholesome foods is learning to savor them by chewing thoroughly. You won't want to waste any enjoyment of this gourmet-quality meal by rushing through it. Chew slowly, and as you do, take time to relish the crunch of the coating on the fish, the tender flakiness of the meat itself, and the contrasting sweet and tart essences of the mango salsa.

Chewing your food thoroughly is also important for health-related reasons. Enzymes in the saliva do the initial work of digesting food while it is still in the mouth. If you swallow too soon, you fail to maximize nutrient absorption and you risk allowing larger food particles to burden the system. Interestingly, thorough chewing has also been associated with better memory, according to researcher Andrew Scholey of the University of Northumbria, in Newcastle, U.K. In the results of a study on chewing and memory published in March 2002, chewing one's food well was associated with an improvement in both long-term and short-term memory.

Chicken Curry Made Simple

PER SERVING: 366.8 CALORIES ~ 34.2 G PROTEIN ~ 12.2 G CARBOHYDRATE ~ 2.2 G FIBER ~ 20.9 G
TOTAL FAT ~ 15.3 G SATURATED FAT ~ 78.8 MG CHOLESTEROL ~ 281.4 MG SODIUM

This recipe comes from my friend Stephanie Findley, of McMinnville, Oregon. It's perfect for those nights when you don't want to spend much time in the kitchen. To make the job even quicker, chop the vegetables ahead of time. Serve over a favorite grain such as aromatic jasmine rice or quinoa.

1 large onion, chopped	2–3 boneless, skinless organic chicken breasts (about 1½ pounds meat), cubed
3–4 cloves garlic, minced	
1 tablespoon olive oil	1 13.5-ounce can coconut milk
5–6 carrots, sliced into sticks	Curry powder to taste
1 14.5-ounce can organic chicken broth	Ginger powder to taste

In a large saucepan, sauté garlic and onions in half of the olive oil over medium heat. Add carrots and continue sautéing.

While carrots are cooking, in a separate saucepan sauté chicken in remaining olive oil until done. To the saucepan with the vegetables, add chicken broth, coconut milk, and cooked chicken. Add curry powder and ginger to taste. (I use 2–4 teaspoons curry powder and 1–2 teaspoons ginger powder.) Continue to cook until flavors meld and sauce is heated through, about 10 minutes.

Serves 5.

Substitutions
You can add any vegetables you like to this versatile recipe. Broccoli always makes a good addition to curries.

Healthy Tidbit
Do not drink anything with your meals. You can drink a small amount of water with apple cider vinegar before a meal, but do not drink anything while you are eating as doing so can dilute your digestive enzymes and decrease digestion. If you must have some fluid with your meals, drink small sips of water occasionally throughout the meal.

Nutritional Analysis per Serving			
Vitamin A	1763.2 RE	Vitamin D	0.0 µg
Thiamin (B-1)	0.1 mg	Vitamin E	0.0 mg
Riboflavin (B-2)	0.2 mg	Calcium	63.1 mg
Niacin	13.3 mg	Iron	3.8 mg
Vitamin B-6	0.8 mg	Phosphorus	400.5 mg
Vitamin B-12	0.3 µg	Magnesium	73.6 mg
Folate (total)	29.8 µg	Zinc	1.7 mg
Vitamin C	7.6 mg	Potassium	763.8 mg

Coconut Almond Chicken

PER SERVING: 505.3 CALORIES ~ 33.0 G PROTEIN ~ 48.4 G CARBOHYDRATE ~ 3.8 G FIBER ~ 21.0 G TOTAL FAT ~ 3.5 G SATURATED FAT ~ 65.7 MG CHOLESTEROL ~ 839.5 MG SODIUM

I converted this recipe from one for peanut sauce. Though the original was meant to be served cold, I prefer it warm. Instead of the rice noodles called for in the recipe, you can serve this rich and hearty dish with just about any grain.

4 green onions, white part only, chopped

4 garlic cloves, minced

2 teaspoons olive oil

½ cup smooth almond butter

1 cup light coconut milk

2 tablespoons fresh lemon juice

2 tablespoons wheat-free tamari

1 tablespoon fish sauce

½ cup water

2–3 boneless, skinless organic chicken breasts (about 1½ pounds meat), cubed

2 heads of broccoli, including the stalk, chopped

½ pound thin rice noodles, cooked according to package directions

¼ cup roasted nuts, for garnish

¼ cup dried cranberries, for garnish

Sauté the garlic and onions in olive oil until softened and slightly brown. In a blender, combine cooked garlic and onions with almond butter, coconut milk, lemon juice, tamari, fish sauce, and water. Blend until smooth.

In a large skillet, combine blended sauce, chicken, and broccoli. Cover and cook until chicken is done, about 15 minutes. Before serving, add cranberries and nuts. Serves 6.

Substitutions

For vegetarians, tofu works well in place of the chicken. For a lower-fat version, substitute an alternative milk (rice, soy, almond) for the coconut milk.

Nutritional Analysis per Serving

Vitamin A	86.4 RE	Vitamin D	0.0 µg
Thiamin (B-1)	0.1 mg	Vitamin E	0.3 mg
Riboflavin (B-2)	0.3 mg	Calcium	115.7 mg
Niacin	11.8 mg	Iron	3.2 mg
Vitamin B-6	0.7 mg	Phosphorus	362.8 mg
Vitamin B-12	0.3 µg	Magnesium	124.5 mg
Folate (total)	64.8 µg	Zinc	2.1 mg
Vitamin C	52.9 mg	Potassium	655.5 mg

Healthy Tidbit

Coconut is a great source of plant-based fat, especially for vegetarians. Be aware that coconut oil is a saturated fat and should therefore be used sparingly if you have poor lipid profiles. Coconut tonifies the heart and has been useful in quenching thirst, supporting diabetes treatment, and decreasing edema. It helps to nurture the body and can increase semen, build up the blood, increase energy, and develop body mass due to its fat content.

Dr. Erika's Quinoa Stir Fry

PER SERVING: 284.3 CALORIES ~ 8.6 G PROTEIN ~ 40.5 G CARBOHYDRATE ~ 7.2 G FIBER ~ 11.6 G
TOTAL FAT ~ 1.5 G SATURATED FAT ~ 0.0 MG CHOLESTEROL ~ 239.5 MG SODIUM

Erika Siegel, N.D., L.Ac., who contributed this recipe, calls this salad a "prescription for nutrients."

It tastes great any time of year, makes tasty leftovers, and can complement most dinners, so be sure to keep it in your repertoire.

⅓ cup quinoa	4 large kale leaves, chopped
⅔ cup plus ½ cup filtered water	2 large carrots, chopped
⅛ teaspoon salt	2 cups chopped broccoli (heads and stem)
1 tablespoon olive oil	
¼ teaspoon mustard seeds	1 teaspoon sesame oil
½ teaspoon whole cumin seeds	Dash of sea salt or wheat-free tamari
1 medium onion, chopped	¼ cup raisins and/or ¼ cup chopped almonds (optional), for garnish

In a small saucepan, bring quinoa, ⅔ cup water, and ⅛ teaspoon salt to a boil. Cover, reduce heat to medium, and simmer for 15 minutes.

In a deep, large pan over medium heat, sauté mustard and cumin seeds in olive oil until mustard seeds pop. Add onions, and sauté on low heat until onions soften.

Immediately add kale, carrots, broccoli, and ½ cup filtered water. Sauté 3–5 minutes on low to medium heat, till the vegetables are crisp-tender. Add remaining ingredients; combine all in a large bowl with cooked quinoa.

Serve warm or cool.

Serves 2.

Substitutions
This recipe works well with many different vegetables, so feel free to improvise based on what is in your refrigerator.

Healthy Tidbit
Mustard seeds stimulate circulation and have been used to treat bronchitis, in poultices, and to reduce inflammation in joints.

Nutritional Analysis per Serving

Vitamin A	2,150.3 RE	Vitamin D	0.0 µg
Thiamin (B-1)	0.2 mg	Vitamin E	0.0 mg
Riboflavin (B-2)	0.3 mg	Calcium	143.0 mg
Niacin	2.4 mg	Iron	4.5 mg
Vitamin B-6	0.5 mg	Phosphorus	235.2 mg
Vitamin B-12	0.0 µg	Magnesium	105.3 mg
Folate (total)	101.4 µg	Zinc	1.7 mg
Vitamin C	125.9 mg	Potassium	924.0 mg

Easy Baked Chicken

PER SERVING: 510.5 CALORIES ~ 56.3 G PROTEIN ~ 46.6 G CARBOHYDRATE ~ 8.4 G FIBER ~ 10.3 G
TOTAL FAT ~ 1.8 G SATURATED FAT ~ 131.4 MG CHOLESTEROL ~ 475.7 MG SODIUM

Pam Quataert brought this dish to a potluck supper. I was so impressed
that I had to include it in this book.

1½ cups organic chicken broth

1 teaspoon dried thyme

1 cup rice wine vinegar

1½ tablespoons miso paste

1 tablespoon garlic powder

1 large onion, sliced

1½ pounds yams, sliced

5 large carrots, quartered, or 25 baby carrots

6–8 organic boneless, skinless chicken breasts (about 3 pounds total)

3 tablespoons olive oil

2 tablespoons dried parsley

Dash cayenne pepper

Preheat oven to 475° F.

In a small mixing bowl, combine chicken broth, thyme, rice wine
vinegar, miso paste, and garlic powder.

Place sliced vegetables in a 13 x 9-inch baking dish. Arrange chicken
breasts on top. Pour broth mixture over the chicken, and sprinkle with
olive oil, parsley, and cayenne pepper.

Bake at 475° F, covered, for 1 hour, or until meat is browned. Turn
the meat once after about 30 minutes. Serve warm with a green salad or
brown rice. Serves 6.

Substitutions

Boneless, skinless organic turkey breast works well, too. Experiment
with other seasonings (e.g.,
rosemary in place of thyme)
and other vegetables. Prepare everything in the
morning or the night
before, so when you get
home from work you can
just preheat the oven and
pop it in.

Nutritional Analysis per Serving

Vitamin A	2,894.1 RE	Vitamin D	0.0 µg
Thiamin (B-1)	0.3 mg	Vitamin E	0.0 mg
Riboflavin (B-2)	0.3 mg	Calcium	97.8 mg
Niacin	22.0 mg	Iron	3.3 mg
Vitamin B-6	1.5 mg	Phosphorus	533.8 mg
Vitamin B-12	0.6 µg	Magnesium	89.5 mg
Folate (total)	51.0 µg	Zinc	2.5 mg
Vitamin C	24.6 mg	Potassium	1,837.4 mg

Healthy Tidbit

One of the most important ways to balance the endocrine system is to establish a regular daily routine, including when you eat, when you get up in the morning, and when you go to sleep. Eating at the same time each day prepares your body for digestion at that time of day. Having a regular sleep-wake cycle helps to balance thyroid and adrenal function.

Falafel Burgers

PER SERVING: 301.9 CALORIES ~ 9.5 G PROTEIN ~ 41.7 G CARBOHYDRATE ~ 7.9 G FIBER ~ 11.8 G
TOTAL FAT ~ 1.6 G SATURATED FAT ~ 0.0 MG CHOLESTEROL ~ 1,090.7 MG SODIUM

These delicious Mediterranean burgers can be served with many different side dishes. This recipe comes from my good friend and colleague Erika Siegel, N.D., L.Ac.

2 tablespoons olive oil

1½ cup minced onions

3 cloves garlic

1 teaspoon ground cumin seeds

1 cup finely chopped carrot

1¾ cup (15-ounce can) cooked chickpeas (garbanzo beans), drained

1½ tablespoons tahini (sesame paste)

¼ cup minced fresh parsley

¹/₃ cup plus 1 tablespoon chickpea flour

½ teaspoon baking soda

1 teaspoon salt

Juice of ½ medium lemon

In a large skillet over medium heat, sauté onions in 1 tablespoon olive oil until soft. Add garlic, cumin, seeds and carrot. Sauté for 2 more minutes. Transfer to a large bowl.

Add drained chickpeas; mash by hand or in a food processor. Add tahini and parsley.

In a smaller bowl, combine chickpea flour, baking soda, and salt. Add to mashed chickpea mixture in large bowl, and mix well. With floured hands, form 4 patties and lightly dust with remaining tablespoon chickpea flour.

Heat 1 tablespoon olive oil in a large skillet over medium heat. Add patties to skillet. After 1 minute, or when browning begins, flip the patties. Cook for about 2 minutes before flipping again. Keep cooking, turning every minute or two, until they are a deep golden brown on both sides.

Squeeze fresh lemon juice on top. Serve immediately with hummus or baba ghanoush.

Serves 4.

Healthy Tidbit

The traditional diets of Mediterranean peoples have been extensively studied in recent years due to the low incidence of

Nutritional Analysis per Serving			
Vitamin A	877.3 RE	Vitamin D	0.0 µg
Thiamin (B-1)	0.2 mg	Vitamin E	0.0 mg
Riboflavin (B-2)	0.1 mg	Calcium	84.7 mg
Niacin	1.1 mg	Iron	3.0 mg
Vitamin B-6	0.7 mg	Phosphorus	204.8 mg
Vitamin B-12	0.0 µg	Magnesium	66.0 mg
Folate (total)	141.1 µg	Zinc	1.9 mg
Vitamin C	21.0 mg	Potassium	523.0 mg

chronic diseases and high life expectancies attributed to these populations. The Mediterranean diet delivers as much as 40 percent of total daily calories from fat, yet the incidence of cardiovascular diseases in some Mediterranean countries is lower than in the U.S. Experts speculate that the difference must be due in part to the type of fat that is consumed: In the traditional Mediterrranean diet, olive oil is used generously, fish is eaten often, and red meat is eaten sparingly.

Leftover Veggie Burgers

This is one of those recipes that always comes through in a pinch. It turns out different every time and transforms your leftovers into something fun to eat. *Note:* We didn't include nutritional information because the point of this recipe is to experiment with whatever leftovers you have on hand.

1 cup leftover cooked vegetables (stir-fried, steamed, etc.)

½ cup leftover cooked brown rice, quinoa, etc., from previous night

2 organic eggs, beaten

½ mashed banana (optional), as a binding agent

Preheat oven to 375° F.

Combine all ingredients in a blender; blend until the vegetables and grains are finely chopped. Form the mixture into patties, and place them on a greased baking pan. Bake until crisp around the edges, about 18 minutes.

Another option is to chop the leftover veggies in a chopper or food processor, and then mix them with the other ingredients in a bowl, using your hands. If you don't have either a chopper or a blender, just mince the vegetables by hand and mix them with the remaining ingredients. You shouldn't need to season the burgers, because your meal from the night before will have already been seasoned.

Serves 2.

Substitutions

You can add so many different things to these burgers. Try tuna fish, cooked beans of any kind, nuts, or seeds. If you cannot tolerate eggs, use another binder from the substitutions table in the Appendix.

Healthy Tidbit

This is a much healthier burger than one containing red meat, which increases levels of arachidonic acid in the body and can lead to inflammation. It is also better for lipid levels and digestive tract health.

Maki-zushi (Sushi Rolls)

PER SERVING: 461.7 CALORIES ~ 9.3 G PROTEIN ~ 92.6 G CARBOHYDRATE ~ 5.8 G FIBER ~ 6.2 G
TOTAL FAT ~ 1.0 G SATURATED FAT ~ 0.0 MG CHOLESTEROL ~ 207.2 MG SODIUM

Restaurant sushi is expensive and often contains sugar in the rice. It is fun and easy to make your own sushi rolls at home. You can do some amazing things with rice and a sheet of toasted seaweed. I use a combination of white and brown rice, upping the nutritional quality, and I usually make vegetarian rolls.

> 2 cups short-grain brown rice
> 1¹/₃ cups short-grain white rice
> 5 cups filtered water
> 4 tablespoons rice vinegar
> ½ tablespoon salt
> 1½ tablespoon maple syrup or brown rice syrup
> 8 sheets toasted seaweed
> 1 cucumber, sliced lengthwise in very thin slices
> 1 carrot, sliced lengthwise in very thin slices
> 1 avocado, sliced lengthwise in very thin slices
> Wheat-free tamari for dipping
> Wasabi paste, to be added as a spice to tamari dipping sauce
> Toasted sesame seeds, to sprinkle on top
> *Special equipment:* 1 sushi roller and paddle (available at Asian grocers for under $5)

Combine rice and water in a medium saucepan, cover, and bring to a boil. Boil for about 2 minutes.

Meanwhile, prepare vinegar mixture by combining vinegar, salt, and sweetener.

Reduce heat to medium, and boil for 5 more minutes. Add the vinegar mixture directly to the rice and water. Then reduce heat to very low and simmer for about 15 minutes or until water has been absorbed.

While rice is cooking, prepare vegetables by cutting them into thin, long strips.

Nutritional Analysis per Serving			
Vitamin A	351.1 RE	Vitamin D	0.0 µg
Thiamin (B-1)	0.4 mg	Vitamin E	0.4 mg
Riboflavin (B-2)	0.1 mg	Calcium	45.8 mg
Niacin	5.2 mg	Iron	3.3 mg
Vitamin B-6	0.5 mg	Phosphorus	229.4 mg
Vitamin B-12	0.0 µg	Magnesium	117.5 mg
Folate (total)	101.3 µg	Zinc	2.3 mg
Vitamin C	6.2 mg	Potassium	447.3 mg

When rice is finished, remove from heat and allow to cool.

Place one sheet of seaweed on sushi roller, making sure to arrange the sheet so that the perforation will aid in cutting the roll once you assemble it. Place the seaweed sheet so the rough side faces up (i.e., will be in contact with the rice).

Spoon a small amount of rice onto seaweed sheet, and pat it flat with the sushi paddle, leaving a border of ½–1 inch without rice at the top edge of the seaweed sheet.

Place 1–2 strips of each vegetable on top of the rice at the bottom edge of the seaweed sheet. Use sushi roller to roll it up, like a jelly roll. With a very sharp, serrated, clean knife, cut the roll into ³/₄-inch maki-zushi, or sushi rolls.

Note: As with anything, learning to make sushi rolls can take a little practice. Your earliest ones will still taste great, however, so use them as "tasters" until you have a better handle on the technique. Helpful hints: Clean the knife between each roll, or dip into water periodically to remove rice buildup. Allow yourself plenty of time to get the feel of it. Sometimes using less rice and fewer vegetables can make it easier to roll.

Sprinkle the rolls with toasted sesame seeds, arrange on a platter, and serve immediately. Each person should get his/her own sauce dish to mix tamari and wasabi to desired taste.

Serves 6.

Substitutions
Sushi rolls are very fun to experiment with. Ideas for veggies include radishes, bok choy, or pickles. Tofu cut into long, thin slices works well. Try adding smoked salmon or sushi-grade raw fish. Or just serve the raw fish over sticky rice. Adding toasted sesame seeds to the rice is another fun idea.

Healthy Tidbit
From a nutritional standpoint it is almost hard to pick out the best characteristics of seaweed, because it contains more vitamins and minerals than any other class of food. It is high in calcium, iodine, phosphorus, sodium, and iron. It is a rich source of protein and of vitamins A, B-complex, C, and E. Due to its iodine content, seaweed can also support thyroid function; it can help to reduce a goiter that is related to hypothyroidism.

Lentil and Nut Loaf

PER SERVING: 541.2 CALORIES ~ 20.6 G PROTEIN ~ 50.1 G CARBOHYDRATE ~ 16.3 G FIBER ~ 31.1 G TOTAL FAT ~ 3.5 G SATURATED FAT ~ 70.5 MG CHOLESTEROL ~ 262.0 MG SODIUM

This is a good vegetarian option for meatloaf. Serve it with roasted vegetables or a salad.

8 ounces dried lentils	2 teaspoons oregano
1 large onion, chopped	3 tablespoons fresh parsley, chopped
8 cloves of garlic, cut in half	2 organic eggs
1 tablespoon extra-virgin olive oil	½ mashed banana
2 cups walnuts, ground	Sea salt to taste
2 cups cooked brown rice	Black pepper to taste
2 tablespoons teriyaki sauce	

Soak lentils for at least 3 hours, and then simmer for 20 minutes or until softened.

Preheat oven to 350° F.

Sauté garlic and onions with olive oil in a small skillet over medium heat for 3–5 minutes. Mix all ingredients together and press into a greased 9 x 5-inch loaf pan.

Bake for 1 hour or until cooked through.

Serves 6.

Substitutions

Experiment with any ground nut or a combination of 2 or 3 types of nuts. In place of the rice, try cooked amaranth, cooked quinoa, or 2 cups nonwheat bread crumbs.

Healthy Tidbit

Beans and legumes strengthen kidneys and adrenal glands, thereby promoting cellular regeneration, physical growth, and elimination. By supporting adrenal function, they help with the stress response, blood sugar regulation, blood pressure regulation, and sex hormone production.

Nutritional Analysis per Serving			
Vitamin A	48.9 RE	Vitamin D	0.2 µg
Thiamin (B-1)	0.5 mg	Vitamin E	0.0 mg
Riboflavin (B-2)	0.2 mg	Calcium	97.4 mg
Niacin	2.4 mg	Iron	4.7 mg
Vitamin B-6	0.6 mg	Phosphorus	402.2 mg
Vitamin B-12	0.2 µg	Magnesium	141.5 mg
Folate (total)	151.2 µg	Zinc	3.6 mg
Vitamin C	97.4 mg	Potassium	607.5 mg

Mung Dal

PER SERVING: 258.5 CALORIES ~ 11.2 G PROTEIN ~ 46.1 G CARBOHYDRATE ~ 11.0 G FIBER ~ 3.2 G TOTAL FAT ~ 0.4 G SATURATED FAT ~ 0.0 MG CHOLESTEROL ~ 202.2 MG SODIUM

Dal is a Hindi word for all types of dried beans, split peas, and lentils. There are many different varieties of dal, all of which have a specific use in Indian cooking. Mung dal is made from the beans of the mung plant. This recipe is from my good friend Chelsea Phillips, MSOM, who is an acupuncturist practicing in Bend, Oregon.

1 tablespoon olive oil

1 tablespoon black mustard seeds

1 bunch green onions, chopped small

1 cup basmati rice

1 cup yellow mung dal (from Indian markets or some health-food stores)

6 cups filtered water

1 large handful cilantro, minced

¼ teaspoon ground cumin

¼ teaspoon coriander

¼ teaspoon turmeric

¼ teaspoon ginger powder

½ teaspoon sea salt

Sauté mustard seeds in olive oil over medium heat until they begin to pop. Add the green onions and sauté until onions are soft.

Rinse and drain rice.

Combine all ingredients, including the sautéed onions and mustard seeds, in a large saucepan.

Bring to a boil, reduce heat to medium-low, cover, and simmer for 25–30 minutes or until rice is cooked.

Serve warm with steamed vegetables or a green salad.

Serves 6.

Substitutions

You may be able to use lentils in place of the mung dal.

Healthy Tidbit

Coriander—and the herb that grows from it, cilantro—is commonly

Nutritional Analysis per Serving			
Vitamin A	13.4 RE	Vitamin D	0.0 µg
Thiamin (B-1)	0.2 mg	Vitamin E	0.0 mg
Riboflavin (B-2)	0.1 mg	Calcium	45.9 mg
Niacin	0.8 mg	Iron	3.2 mg
Vitamin B-6	0.1 mg	Phosphorus	144.5 mg
Vitamin B-12	0.0 µg	Magnesium	37.6 mg
Folate (total)	95.9 µg	Zinc	1.5 mg
Vitamin C	7.0 mg	Potassium	329.8 mg

used in Middle Eastern and Asian cooking. The Egyptians used it as an aphrodisiac and the Greeks used it to flavor their wines. Coriander is a mild sedative, aids digestion, reduces gas and bloating, and eases migraines. The essential oil is used in massage oils and may be helpful for cramps and facial neuralgia.

Cold Asian Noodles with Smoked Salmon

PER SERVING: 669.7 CALORIES ~ 17.8 G PROTEIN ~ 110.0 G CARBOHYDRATE ~ 3.4 G FIBER ~ 17.0
G TOTAL FAT ~ 2.7 G SATURATED FAT ~ 13.0 MG CHOLESTEROL ~ 1,690.7 MG SODIUM

Even though this is a salad, my family loves it for dinner. It is large
enough to feed two as a main course; if you are feeding more, double the
recipe.

8 ounces rice noodles

1 cucumber, peeled and cut into thin strips

1 yellow pepper, cut into thin strips

4 ounces smoked salmon, sliced (try to get salmon with no nitrites,
preservatives, or added colors)

3–4 tablespoon teriyaki sauce

2 tablespoons rice vinegar

2 tablespoons toasted sesame oil

2 tablespoons toasted sesame seeds, for garnish

Cook rice noodles according to package directions. I usually bring a pot
of water to boil, add the noodles, turn off the burner, and let them cook
for 5–7 minutes until they reach the desired texture.

Slice the cucumber, yellow pepper, and salmon while the noodles are
softening.

Whisk together the teriyaki sauce, rice vinegar, and sesame oil.
When the noodles are finished, rinse them with cold water, and toss
them with the dressing.

In a large serving bowl, combine noodles with cucumber, yellow
pepper, and salmon.

Garnish with sesame seeds and serve chilled.

Serves 2.

Substitutions
Try cooked chicken instead of smoked salmon. Try red pepper, radishes,
or carrots in place of yellow pepper.

Healthy Tidbit
Salmon is a wonderful
source of omega-3 essential
fatty acids, which makes it
the ideal food for the anti-
inflammatory diet (omega-3

Nutritional Analysis per Serving			
Vitamin A	68.7 RE	Vitamin D	0.0 µg
Thiamin (B-1)	0.1 mg	Vitamin E	0.0 mg
Riboflavin (B-2)	0.2 mg	Calcium	67.7 mg
Niacin	4.2 mg	Iron	2.6 mg
Vitamin B-6	0.4 mg	Phosphorus	366.5 mg
Vitamin B-12	1.8 µg	Magnesium	71.0 mg
Folate (total)	44.7 µg	Zinc	1.5 mg
Vitamin C	174.9 mg	Potassium	612.4 mg

fatty acids help to reduce inflammation). Salmon that is harvested from the wild offers the highest content of essential fatty acids. Farm-raised salmon contain fewer fatty acids, and the fish are given feed that has been dyed to give their flesh the pink color that occurs naturally in wild salmon. Whenever possible, buy wild salmon. You will notice a difference in taste, and your body will benefit from the higher quality of the nutrients.

Pesto Pizza with Chicken

PER SERVING: 277.8 CALORIES ~ 15.9 G PROTEIN ~ 5.4 G CARBOHYDRATE ~ 1.6 G FIBER ~ 22.0 G
TOTAL FAT ~ 3.0 G SATURATED FAT ~ 34.2 MG CHOLESTEROL ~ 178.9 MG SODIUM

It may seem impossible to make an anti-inflammatory pizza, but this recipe does the trick.

For the crust, follow the Spelt Bread recipe on page 93 (for two pizza crusts, make one recipe)

2 cups Basil Pesto (see recipe on page 59)	VeganRella cheese substitute, grated (optional)
1 tablespoon olive oil	¼ cup cashews, ground
3 cloves garlic, minced	Vegetables, chopped (optional)
1 medium onion, chopped	Sea salt to taste
2 organic chicken breasts, cubed	Pepper to taste
1 teaspoon dried basil	
1 teaspoon dried oregano	

Make dough as instructed in the spelt bread recipe.

Prepare pesto (or defrost a jar of homemade pesto).

Heat olive oil in a skillet over medium heat. Add garlic, onion, chicken, basil, oregano, and any vegetables you want to include. Cook until chicken is nearly done and vegetables are crisp-tender, about 10 minutes.

After dough has risen, preheat oven to 400° F. Divide the dough in half and stretch flat onto two generously greased pizza pans.

Cover the dough with pesto, and top with sautéed onions, garlic, and chicken, making sure to spread evenly. Then, sprinkle with sea salt and pepper if desired. Finish with an even layer of grated cheese substitute.

Bake for 15–20 minutes or until crust is browned.

Remove from oven, allow to cool slightly, and serve with ground cashews sprinkled on top. You'll never know you're not eating parmesan.

Serves 8.

Substitutions

Many cheese substitutes contain small amounts of dairy, so not just any substitute can be used. This recipe is very tasty even without the cheese substi-

Nutritional Analysis per Serving			
Vitamin A	87.6 RE	Vitamin D	0.0 µg
Thiamin (B-1)	0.1 mg	Vitamin E	0.0 mg
Riboflavin (B-2)	0.1 mg	Calcium	55.6 mg
Niacin	5.8 mg	Iron	1.9 mg
Vitamin B-6	0.4 mg	Phosphorus	169.4 mg
Vitamin B-12	0.1 µg	Magnesium	58.2 mg
Folate (total)	23.6 µg	Zinc	1.3 mg
Vitamin C	6.2 mg	Potassium	314.8 mg

tute, especially when you top it with ground cashews. Vary your other toppings according to taste and availability.

Healthy Tidbit
Basil helps to restore balance to the lung and stomach meridians; therefore, it can help with complaints related to those bodily systems. It calms the nerves, aids digestion, and has antibacterial and antiparasitic properties.

Mezza Luna Pizzeria's Pizza Sauce

PER SERVING: 184.4 CALORIES ~ 2.8 G PROTEIN ~ 13.3 G CARBOHYDRATE ~ 0.6 G FIBER ~ 14.7 G
TOTAL FAT ~ 2.5 G SATURATED FAT ~ 0.0 MG CHOLESTEROL ~ 274.0 MG SODIUM

Mezza Luna Pizzeria, located in Eugene, Oregon, offers a tasty option for a tomato-free sauce. Follow the recipe instructions for pesto pizza with chicken (on the previous page), and just use this sauce in place of the pesto.

1½ cups roasted red peppers (you can purchase them in a jar already roasted) *or* 2 large red bell peppers, roasted, peeled, and seeded

½ cup cashews (dry roasted, unsalted)

3 cloves roasted garlic

2 tablespoons olive oil

¼ teaspoon sea salt

¼ teaspoon black pepper

Place all ingredients in a food processor or blender and process until smooth. Makes enough for a single 18-inch pizza or 2 smaller pizzas.
Serves 4.

Substitutions
Top with any vegetables you want, and even try it without the cheese substitute.

Healthy Tidbit
In the September 2005 issue of the journal *Circulation,* the American Heart Association published new guidelines on diet and lifestyle to aid in the prevention of heart disease. General dietary recommendations for children age 2 years and older stress fruits and vegetables, whole grains, low-fat and nonfat dairy products, beans, fish, and lean meat, balanced with sixty minutes of strenuous exercise or play daily. The guidelines recommended for adults include lowering intake of trans and saturated fats, dietary cholesterol, and added sugar and salt; participating in regular physical activity; and maintaining a normal weight for height. This recipe for pizza sauce meets the dietary recommendations for both kids and adults, as well as avoiding the potentially inflammatory effects of tomatoes.

Nutritional Analysis per Serving

Vitamin A	170.9 RE	Vitamin D	0.0 µg
Thiamin (B-1)	0.0 mg	Vitamin E	0.0 mg
Riboflavin (B-2)	0.0 mg	Calcium	12.5 mg
Niacin	0.3 mg	Iron	1.1 mg
Vitamin B-6	0.1 mg	Phosphorus	87.6 mg
Vitamin B-12	0.0 µg	Magnesium	45.3 mg
Folate (total)	11.9 µg	Zinc	1.0 mg
Vitamin C	0.7 mg	Potassium	107.5 mg

Seared Tuna over Raw Vegetables

PER SERVING: 195.3 CALORIES ~ 28.9 G PROTEIN ~ 6.8 G CARBOHYDRATE ~ 2.3 G FIBER ~ 5.6 G
TOTAL FAT ~ 0.9 G SATURATED FAT ~ 50.6 MG CHOLESTEROL ~ 582.8 MG SODIUM

Many fish lovers agree that the best way to enjoy high-quality tuna is served rare. However, if you have a difficult time eating partially raw fish, you can bake or sear the tuna for this recipe until it is cooked all the way through.

10 radishes, grated

3 large carrots, grated

½ cup chopped cabbage

2 fillets of yellow fin tuna, sushi-grade if possible (about 1 pound of meat total)

2 teaspoons olive oil

2 tablespoons wheat-free tamari (for dipping)

¼ teaspoon wasabi paste (optional)

2 tablespoons toasted sesame seeds

Combine radishes, carrots, and cabbage in a large serving bowl.

Heat olive oil in a medium skillet over high heat until oil is shimmering but not smoking. Cook the tuna fillets on one side for about 3 minutes, until they develop a thin (3-millimeter) layer of white, cooked flesh. Turn fillets over, and sear for another 3 minutes or so until they develop a white, cooked layer on that side. The fillets' centers will still be pink.

Remove fillets from heat and slice lengthwise into thin slices; make sure each piece has pink in the center and white around the edge.

Arrange the seared tuna slices on top of the grated vegetables; garnish with toasted sesame seeds. Serve with tamari and wasabi for dipping. Serves 4.

Substitutions

Another option is to serve the tuna over sticky rice, prepared as you would for the Maki-zushi recipe (see page 141). You can use teriyaki sauce instead of tamari for dipping, but make sure it doesn't contain added sugar or wheat.

Nutritional Analysis per Serving			
Vitamin A	1,306.6 RE	Vitamin D	0.0 µg
Thiamin (B-1)	0.5 mg	Vitamin E	0.0 mg
Riboflavin (B-2)	0.1 mg	Calcium	85.9 mg
Niacin	12.2 mg	Iron	1.9 mg
Vitamin B-6	1.1 mg	Phosphorus	276.9 mg
Vitamin B-12	0.6 µg	Magnesium	84.0 mg
Folate (total)	23.4 µg	Zinc	1.1 mg
Vitamin C	8.1 mg	Potassium	737.7 mg

Healthy Tidbit

Radishes stimulate the appetite and aid in digestion; they can be beneficial if eaten before or after a meal. Radishes are also antibacterial and antifungal. Radish sprouts, which can be grown in 4 days, lend a spicy hint to salads and stir-fries.

Stuffed Chicken Breast with "Peanut" Curry Sauce

PER SERVING: 633.5 CALORIES ~ 46.5 G PROTEIN ~ 34.9 G CARBOHYDRATE ~ 2.7 G FIBER ~ 35.8 G TOTAL FAT ~ 20.3 G SATURATED FAT ~ 98.6 MG CHOLESTEROL ~ 704.6 MG SODIUM

I invented this dish one night when I was having a friend over for dinner. I was late getting home, my daughter needed attention, and I felt as if I had nothing to cook. I had some leftover lemon vegetable rice, and I decided to stuff it into chicken breasts and make a sauce for it. It turned out great—like I had been slaving in the kitchen for hours. For the side dish, I drizzled the same sauce over steamed green beans, which were the only vegetables I had in the refrigerator. No extra work!

4 organic boneless, skinless chicken breasts, about 6 ounces each, sliced lengthwise to form a pocket almost as large as the chicken breast (leave about ¼ inch uncut at both ends)

2 cups leftover Lemon Vegetable Rice (see recipe on page 66)

For the sauce
4–5 garlic cloves, minced
1 tablespoon olive oil (for sautéing)
1 13.5-ounce can coconut milk
2 tablespoons almond butter
4 teaspoons curry powder
1 tablespoon wheat-free tamari
1 teaspoon fish sauce
2 teaspoons honey or maple syrup

Preheat oven to 400° F.

After cutting chicken breasts to form pockets, stuff them generously with ¼–½ cup of the lemon rice. Bake for 25–30 minutes or until chicken is finished cooking.

For the sauce, in a 2-quart saucepan over medium heat, sauté garlic in olive oil. When garlic is soft, stir in the other ingredients. Bring to a simmer, then reduce heat to low. To allow the flavors to blend, continue cooking, stirring occasionally, until chicken is done.

Once chicken is finished, pour sauce over the breasts and serve warm.

Serves 4.

Substitutions

You can stuff the chicken breasts with any leftover flavored rice, grain, or legume.

Nutritional Analysis per Serving			
Vitamin A	47.8 RE	Vitamin D	0.0 µg
Thiamin (B-1)	0.2 mg	Vitamin E	0.4 mg
Riboflavin (B-2)	0.3 mg	Calcium	100.0 mg
Niacin	17.8 mg	Iron	6.4 mg
Vitamin B-6	1.1 mg	Phosphorus	563.6 mg
Vitamin B-12	0.4 µg	Magnesium	166.5 mg
Folate (total)	45.0 µg	Zinc	3.2 mg
Vitamin C	13.6 mg	Potassium	929.7 mg

Healthy Tidbit

When you sit down to any meal it is important to take a moment and give thanks to the Mother Earth (or to God, the Buddha, the All-That-Is, or your spiritual higher power) for supplying you with the nutrient-filled food you are about to eat. Give thanks for all the plants, animals, and humans who were involved in bringing you the meal—for the chicken, the rice plants and olive trees, the many farmers and distributors along the way. Also give thanks for the friends and family who are dining with you. Give thanks for your health, for the health of your family and friends, and for the willpower to eat well and remain healthy.

Sweet Sprout Curry

PER SERVING: 214.0 CALORIES ~ 5.2 G PROTEIN ~ 43.7 G CARBOHYDRATE ~ 7.5 G FIBER ~ 4.4 G
TOTAL FAT ~ 0.6 G SATURATED FAT ~ 0.0 MG CHOLESTEROL ~ 870.0 MG SODIUM

I love to grow sprouts with the anticipation of this dish in mind. Please see page 170 for instructions on how to grow your own sprouts.

1 onion, minced

1 tablespoon cold-pressed, extra-virgin olive oil

4 carrots, sliced

1 apple, peeled and minced

½ cup raisins (omit if you are diabetic)

1 can organic chicken broth

2 tablespoons spelt flour

1 teaspoon sea salt

1 teaspoon curry powder

¼ teaspoon paprika

2 cups mung bean sprouts

2 cups alfalfa sprouts

In a medium saucepan, sauté onion in olive oil over medium heat until soft. Add all remaining ingredients except the sprouts; simmer until carrots are soft but still have a little crunch.

Add the sprouts and simmer a little longer until sprouts soften but still have a crunchy consistency. Serve immediately.

Serves 4.

Substitutions
Any type of sprouts can be used for this recipe (see pages 170–171 for some ideas). This combination is just my favorite. You can also use any type of nongluten flour without changing the taste. If you are able to tolerate tomatoes, this dish is great with a can of crushed tomatoes instead of organic chicken broth.

Healthy Tidbit
According to "The Fires Within," an article published in the February 23, 2004, issue of *Time* magazine, recent research has been dedicated to the role of inflammation in certain

Nutritional Analysis per Serving			
Vitamin A	3,480.2 RE	Vitamin D	0.0 µg
Thiamin (B-1)	0.2 mg	Vitamin E	0.1 mg
Riboflavin (B-2)	0.2 mg	Calcium	82.1 mg
Niacin	2.0 mg	Iron	1.9 mg
Vitamin B-6	0.3 mg	Phosphorus	221.3 mg
Vitamin B-12	0.0 µg	Magnesium	42.5 mg
Folate (total)	68.9 µg	Zinc	0.8 mg
Vitamin C	19.4 mg	Potassium	840.5 mg

diseases such as Alzheimer's disease, cardiovascular disease, colon cancer, and autoimmune disorders. For example, doctors are finding a connection between inflammation and increased incidence of cardiovascular disease through an inflammatory marker called CRP (C-reactive protein). Instead of taking aspirin or other anti-inflammatory medication for prevention of chronic disease, which can cause harm when used for the long term, try eating healthier instead. Fresh sprouts, which contain lots of fiber and nutrients, are an excellent choice of a food to eat more of in your quest to improve your diet.

Thai Red Curry

PER SERVING: 263.8 CALORIES ~ 6.5 G PROTEIN ~ 31.1 G CARBOHYDRATE ~ 4.4 G FIBER ~ 14.6 G
TOTAL FAT ~ 12.2 G SATURATED FAT ~ 0.0 MG CHOLESTEROL ~ 448.5 MG SODIUM

Curry is one of my favorite dishes; using red curry paste adds a zesty punch. This recipe comes from my good friend and colleague Dr. Matt Fisel. Prepare this restaurant-quality dish whenever you want to impress a dinner guest.

1 13.5-ounce can coconut milk

2 tablespoons Thai red curry paste

1 onion, chopped

4 kaffir lime leaves (find at a Thai or Asian market)

6 ounces raw pumpkin, chopped

5 ounces green beans, chopped

1 red bell pepper, cut into strips

3 small zucchinis, chopped

7-ounce can bamboo tips or shoots, drained and, if desired, sliced in half

2 tablespoons fresh basil leaves, whole or cut in halves

2 tablespoons lemon juice

2 teaspoons brown rice syrup

2 cups cooked brown rice

Combine coconut milk, curry paste, and ½ cup filtered water in a large wok or saucepan. Bring to a boil, stirring occasionally.

Add onion and lime leaves and allow to boil for 3 minutes.

Add pumpkin to the wok and simmer over medium heat for 8 minutes, or until nearly cooked.

Add beans, red bell pepper, and zucchini, and simmer for another 5 minutes. Add water if the sauce is too thick.

Add bamboo shoots and basil and continue cooking until they are warmed.

Add the lemon juice and brown rice syrup; taste, and adjust seasoning as necessary. Serve over brown rice.

Serves 6.

Nutritional Analysis per Serving			
Vitamin A	211.6 RE	Vitamin D	0.0 µg
Thiamin (B-1)	0.2 mg	Vitamin E	0.0 mg
Riboflavin (B-2)	0.2 mg	Calcium	57.4 mg
Niacin	2.5 mg	Iron	3.9 mg
Vitamin B-6	0.5 mg	Phosphorus	193.0 mg
Vitamin B-12	0.0 µg	Magnesium	89.7 mg
Folate (total)	62.2 µg	Zinc	1.5 mg
Vitamin C	65.4 mg	Potassium	677.3 mg

Substitutions

You can make this dish without the lime leaves, but they do add a distinctive flavor. You can also use different vegetables—whatever you have in your crisper drawer. To reduce the spiciness of the dish, reduce the amount of red curry paste you use.

Healthy Tidbit

Pumpkin is usually known only for pies and seeds, but it can be great in many dishes. A very tasty source of vitamins and minerals, pumpkin's nutritious orange flesh offers beta-carotene, potassium, pro-vitamin A, vitamin C, and dietary fiber. Pumpkin seeds and pumpkin seed oil contain zinc and unsaturated fatty acids that are effective in helping prostate problems.

Simple Stir Fry

PER SERVING: 112.8 CALORIES ~ 2.9 G PROTEIN ~ 11.0 G CARBOHYDRATE ~ 2.9 G FIBER ~ 7.0 G
TOTAL FAT ~ 1.0 G SATURATED FAT ~ 0.0 MG CHOLESTEROL ~ 544.7 MG SODIUM

This is the easiest, most basic stir-fry you can fix. If you feel like experimenting with the foods in your refrigerator, this is a great place to start; the vegetables I've listed here are just some ideas. Get creative and be bold with your food choices. See the note below for some tips on selecting veggies for a stir-fry.

2 tablespoons olive oil

2 garlic cloves, minced

1 medium onion, minced

1 cup zucchini, sliced

3 large carrots, sliced

8 crimini mushrooms, sliced

1 large green pepper, chopped

2 tablespoons wheat-free tamari

Sea salt and pepper to taste

Other seasonings to taste (see below)

Sauté garlic and onion in olive oil over medium-high heat until softened.

Add other vegetables and seasonings; cook, stirring often, until vegetables are crisp-tender.

Serves 4.

Note: All stir-fries can begin tasting the same. That's why it's important to get to know your vegetables and seasonings first. Start with a simple stir-fry containing one or two vegetables and one or two seasonings. Practice with the same combination until you have perfected it.

Substitutions
Ideas for seasonings:

— Red pepper flakes

— Dried basil

— Toasted sesame oil (1 tablespoon added at the end of cooking for a nutty Asian flavor)

— Curry paste (1 teaspoon)

Nutritional Analysis per Serving			
Vitamin A	1,315.4 RE	Vitamin D	0.0 µg
Thiamin (B-1)	0.1 mg	Vitamin E	0.0 mg
Riboflavin (B-2)	0.1 mg	Calcium	32.9 mg
Niacin	1.1 mg	Iron	0.8 mg
Vitamin B-6	0.3 mg	Phosphorus	54.1 mg
Vitamin B-12	0.0 µg	Magnesium	20.0 mg
Folate (total)	27.1 µg	Zinc	0.3 mg
Vitamin C	33.6 mg	Potassium	337.2 mg

— Milk Thistle Seasoning Salt (see page 70)

— Nuts for garnish, ground or whole

If you include hearty greens such as kale, chard, etc., add a little water to steam them

Healthy Tidbit

Members of the allium family—onions, garlic, and leeks—all contain a phytochemical that affords protection from cancer. Onions are antiviral and antiseptic. They should be included in the diet often, especially if you are feeling ill or are fighting cancer. Members of the allium family also help to decrease the tendency for clots to form, help to lower LDL cholesterol, and help to decrease total cholesterol—all cardiovascular risk factors. Garlic, onions, and leeks are very versatile. Eat them raw, braised, boiled, steamed, baked, sautéed, scalloped, or grilled.

Turkey Meatloaf

PER SERVING: 217.3 CALORIES ~ 22.5 G PROTEIN ~ 6.1 G CARBOHYDRATE ~ 1.3 G FIBER ~ 11.1 G
TOTAL FAT ~ 3.0 G SATURATED FAT ~ 11.1 MG CHOLESTEROL ~ 415.1 MG SODIUM

This recipe requires little preparation time but needs an hour to bake. It is simple enough to prepare in the morning and throw in the oven as soon as you get home from work. I adapted this recipe from one of my favorite cookbooks, *The Complete Food Allergy Cookbook,* by Marilyn Gioannini, M.D.

1 pound ground organic turkey

¼ cup milk substitute (or chicken or vegetable broth)

1 organic egg

½ cup finely chopped onion

½ cup grated carrot

½ cup minced parsley or cilantro

¼ cup finely chopped celery

½–1½ teaspoon onion powder

½–1½ teaspoon garlic powder

½–1½ teaspoon dried oregano

½–1½ teaspoon dried sage

½ teaspoon salt

¼–½ teaspoon pepper

Preheat oven to 350° F.

Mix all ingredients in a bowl, making sure to blend well. (I use my hands because that's the most effective way to get everything well blended, so dive in and have fun.)

Pat mixture into a greased 9 x 5-inch loaf pan.

Bake for 1 hour. Drain juices and serve by the slice. Kids will love it. Serves 4.

Substitutions

The quantities of spices are given in ranges because some people prefer a more flavorful meatloaf; in that case use the larger quantity. If you cannot tolerate eggs, just replace the egg with ½

Nutritional Analysis per Serving			
Vitamin A	494.8 RE	Vitamin D	0.2 µg
Thiamin (B-1)	0.1 mg	Vitamin E	0.0 mg
Riboflavin (B-2)	0.2 mg	Calcium	57.6 mg
Niacin	3.9 mg	Iron	2.4 mg
Vitamin B-6	0.4 mg	Phosphorus	191.6 mg
Vitamin B-12	0.4 µg	Magnesium	31.3 mg
Folate (total)	34.4 µg	Zinc	2.6 mg
Vitamin C	12.8 mg	Potassium	382.8 mg

banana or other binder. Also add ground or whole flaxseeds, pumpkin seeds, or sunflower seeds.

Healthy Tidbit
Sage is anti-inflammatory, antiseptic, antimicrobial, antifungal, and anti-spasmodic. It can also act as a mild diuretic, act as an astringent, and stimulate the immune system. It stimulates the adrenals, greatly alleviating stress. Clary sage has been used for meditation and spiritual communication. The ancients considered it an oil of protection and psychic sight. It is used to bless a house or a person to keep him or her safe and grounded.

Grains

Amaranth

PER SERVING: 182.3 CALORIES ~ 7.0 G PROTEIN ~ 32.3 G CARBOHYDRATE ~ 4.5 G FIBER ~ 3.2 G
TOTAL FAT ~ 0.8 G SATURATED FAT ~ 0.0 MG CHOLESTEROL ~ 10.2 MG SODIUM

Amaranth does not contain any gluten and thus is recommended for people who can't tolerate that protein. It is rich in lysine, an essential amino acid that many grains lack.

1 cup amaranth

1½ cups filtered water

Place water and amaranth in a 2-quart saucepan. Bring to boil, reduce heat to low, cover, and simmer for 20–25 minutes. Yields 2 cups. Serves 4.

Nutritional Analysis per Serving

Vitamin A	0.0 RE	Vitamin D	0.0 µg
Thiamin (B-1)	0.0 mg	Vitamin E	0.0 mg
Riboflavin (B-2)	0.1 mg	Calcium	74.6 mg
Niacin	0.6 mg	Iron	3.7 mg
Vitamin B-6	0.1 mg	Phosphorus	221.8 mg
Vitamin B-12	0.0 µg	Magnesium	129.7 mg
Folate (total)	23.9 µg	Zinc	1.6 mg
Vitamin C	2.0 mg	Potassium	178.4 mg

Barley

PER SERVING: 93.1 CALORIES ~ 3.3 G PROTEIN ~ 19.3 G CARBOHYDRATE ~ 4.5 G FIBER ~ 0.6 G
TOTAL FAT ~ 0.1 G SATURATED FAT ~ 0.0 MG CHOLESTEROL ~ 3.2 MG SODIUM

Barley has a really good texture for soups and cereal. Buy nonpearled (unhulled) barley because pearling removes more than 30 percent of the grain's nutrition.

1 cup barley

3 cups filtered water

Place water and barley in a 2-quart saucepan. Bring to boil, reduce heat to low, cover, and simmer for 1 hour and 15 minutes. Alternatively, place all ingredients in a crockpot and simmer on high for about 3 hours. Yields 3½ cups. Serves 7.

You can grind your own flour from barley, which can be used to make gravies or can be added to other flours to make baked goods and breads.

Nutritional Analysis per Serving

Vitamin A	0.5 RE	Vitamin D	0.0 µg
Thiamin (B-1)	0.2 mg	Vitamin E	0.0 mg
Riboflavin (B-2)	0.1 mg	Calcium	8.7 mg
Niacin	1.2 mg	Iron	0.9 mg
Vitamin B-6	0.1 mg	Phosphorus	69.4 mg
Vitamin B-12	0.0 µg	Magnesium	35.0 mg
Folate (total)	5.0 µg	Zinc	0.7 mg
Vitamin C	0.0 mg	Potassium	118.8 mg

Brown Rice

PER SERVING: 114.1 CALORIES ~ 2.4 G PROTEIN ~ 23.8 G CARBOHYDRATE ~ 1.1 G FIBER ~ 0.9 G TOTAL FAT ~ 0.2 G SATURATED FAT ~ 0.0 MG CHOLESTEROL ~ 2.2 MG SODIUM

I often use organic short-grain brown rice because it cooks faster and I prefer the texture. Brown rice is superior to white rice in many ways. It has 12 percent more protein, 33 percent more calcium, more B vitamins, and more of other nutrients. I only use white rice for one dish: sushi. Brown rice can complement most dinners and it is good for breakfast. You can also add cooked brown rice to baked goods for extra texture, flavor, and moisture.

1 cup brown rice, short or long grain

2 cups filtered water

Place water and rice in a 2-quart saucepan. Bring to boil; immediately reduce heat to low. Simmer, covered, for 30–40 minutes or until all water has been absorbed. Yields 3 cups. Serves 6.

Nutritional Analysis per Serving

Vitamin A	0.0 RE	Vitamin D	0.0 µg
Thiamin (B-1)	0.1 mg	Vitamin E	0.0 mg
Riboflavin (B-2)	0.0 mg	Calcium	7.1 mg
Niacin	1.6 mg	Iron	0.4 mg
Vitamin B-6	0.1 mg	Phosphorus	97.5 mg
Vitamin B-12	0.0 µg	Magnesium	44.1 mg
Folate (total)	4.3 µg	Zinc	0.6 mg
Vitamin C	0.0 mg	Potassium	65.3 mg

Millet

PER SERVING: 108.0 CALORIES ~ 3.1 G PROTEIN ~ 20.8 G CARBOHYDRATE ~ 2.4 G FIBER ~ 1.2 G TOTAL FAT ~ 0.2 G SATURATED FAT ~ 0.0 MG CHOLESTEROL ~ 1.4 MG SODIUM

Millet can be used in place of rice or quinoa. It adds a crunchy texture to salads and vegetable dishes.

1 cup millet

3 cups filtered water

Place water and millet in a 2-quart saucepan. Bring to boil, reduce heat to low, cover, and simmer for 35–40 minutes. Yields 3½ cups. Serves 7.

Nutritional Analysis per Serving

Vitamin A	0.0 RE	Vitamin D	0.0 µg
Thiamin (B-1)	0.1 mg	Vitamin E	0.0 mg
Riboflavin (B-2)	0.1 mg	Calcium	2.3 mg
Niacin	1.3 mg	Iron	0.9 mg
Vitamin B-6	0.1 mg	Phosphorus	81.4 mg
Vitamin B-12	0.0 µg	Magnesium	32.6 mg
Folate (total)	24.3 µg	Zinc	0.5 mg
Vitamin C	0.0 mg	Potassium	55.7 mg

Oats

PER SERVING: 202.3 CALORIES ~ 8.8 G PROTEIN ~ 34.5 G CARBOHYDRATE ~ 5.5 G FIBER ~ 3.6 G
TOTAL FAT ~ 0.6 G SATURATED FAT ~ 0.0 MG CHOLESTEROL ~ 1.0 MG SODIUM

Oats are sadly underused. Don't just think of them as oatmeal. You can add them to soups and casseroles for a little extra body, or to cookies or other baked goods.

1 cup oats

2 cups filtered water

Place water and oats in a 2-quart saucepan. Cook over low heat for 20–25 minutes. Yields 1³/₄ cups. Serves 3.

Nutritional Analysis per Serving

Vitamin A	0.0 RE	Vitamin D	0.0 µg
Thiamin (B-1)	0.4 mg	Vitamin E	0.0 mg
Riboflavin (B-2)	0.1 mg	Calcium	28.1 mg
Niacin	0.5 mg	Iron	2.5 mg
Vitamin B-6	0.1 mg	Phosphorus	272.0 mg
Vitamin B-12	0.0 µg	Magnesium	92.0 mg
Folate (total)	29.1 µg	Zinc	2.1 mg
Vitamin C	0.0 mg	Potassium	223.1 mg

Quinoa

PER SERVING: 127.2 CALORIES ~ 4.5 G PROTEIN ~ 23.4 G CARBOHYDRATE ~ 2.0 G FIBER ~ 2.0 G
TOTAL FAT ~ 0.2 G SATURATED FAT ~ 0.0 MG CHOLESTEROL ~ 7.1 MG SODIUM

One of my favorite grains, quinoa is very low in gluten. It complements many salads, stir-fries, burgers, egg dishes, meat dishes—just about anything. It is higher in protein than any other grain, and its protein is a complete protein, meaning it contains all of the essential amino acids, a quality shared by very few plant-based foods.

1 cup quinoa

2 cups filtered water

Place water and quinoa in a 2-quart saucepan. Bring to boil and then immediately reduce heat to low. Simmer, covered, for 10–15 minutes or until all water has been absorbed. Yields 2½ cups. Serves 5.

Nutritional Analysis per Serving

Vitamin A	0.0 RE	Vitamin D	0.0 µg
Thiamin (B-1)	0.1 mg	Vitamin E	0.0 mg
Riboflavin (B-2)	0.1 mg	Calcium	20.4 mg
Niacin	1.0 mg	Iron	3.1 mg
Vitamin B-6	0.1 mg	Phosphorus	139.4 mg
Vitamin B-12	0.0 µg	Magnesium	71.4 mg
Folate (total)	16.7 µg	Zinc	1.1 mg
Vitamin C	0.0 mg	Potassium	251.6 mg

Salads

Avocado Bean Salad

PER SERVING: 476.9 CALORIES ~ 9.2 G PROTEIN ~ 37.5 G CARBOHYDRATE ~ 12.1 G FIBER ~ 34.1 G
TOTAL FAT ~ 4.7 G SATURATED FAT ~ 0.0 MG CHOLESTEROL ~ 8.3 MG SODIUM

Avocados are a favorite of mine. The beans give this salad added protein and terrific flavor. Try this recipe for a light but filling lunch.

For the salad:

2 large ripe avocados, peeled and cut into ½ inch cubes

3 cups cooked beans (I like to use 3 different kinds of beans, e.g., pinto, black, kidney, green, garbanzo, others)

½ cup chopped green pepper

½ cup chopped red pepper

6 large lettuce leaves (for serving)

For the dressing:

²/₃ cup olive oil

²/₃ cup rice vinegar

3 tablespoons raw honey

2 teaspoons chopped fresh parsley, divided

2 teaspoons chopped fresh coriander leaves (cilantro)

½ teaspoon black pepper

Combine avocados, beans, and peppers in a bowl.

In a separate bowl, mix dressing ingredients together, leaving half of the parsley for garnish. Carefully coat bean mixture with dressing. Arrange salad on top of lettuce leaves on serving plates.

Sprinkle with reserved parsley and serve immediately.

Serves 6.

Substitutions

Besides experimenting with different beans, you could add many vegetables to this salad. Try artichoke hearts, grated carrots or radishes, or anything else you have in your refrigerator.

Nutritional Analysis per Serving

Vitamin A	122.7 RE	Vitamin D	0.0 µg
Thiamin (B-1)	0.2 mg	Vitamin E	3.8 mg
Riboflavin (B-2)	0.2 mg	Calcium	56.4 mg
Niacin	2.7 mg	Iron	2.7 mg
Vitamin B-6	0.4 mg	Phosphorus	164.3 mg
Vitamin B-12	0.0 µg	Magnesium	63.7 mg
Folate (total)	189.9 µg	Zinc	1.3 mg
Vitamin C	40.9 mg	Potassium	723.4 mg

Healthy Tidbit

We should include at least some raw foods in our diets, because raw vegetables and fruits contain enzymes that may be destroyed in the cooking process. However, if you are in poor health or have compromised digestion, you should eat steamed or cooked vegetables until your health has improved. A good ratio of steamed to raw vegetables for those with satisfactory digestion is 80 percent steamed to 20 percent raw. This also depends on the season. For example, in the summer you are able to digest more fresh and raw foods than in the winter, when digestion slows down.

Many important vitamins and minerals can be lost in the cooking and processing of foods. Vitamin C, for example, is especially vulnerable to destruction by exposure to heat. Raw plant foods such as green leafy vegetables, almonds, pumpkin seeds, and fruits such as avocado can provide essential proteins, essential fatty acids, minerals, and antioxidants often missing from grains.

Home-Grown Alfalfa Sprouts

PER SERVING: 9.6 CALORIES ~ 1.3 G PROTEIN ~ 1.2 G CARBOHYDRATE ~ 0.9 G FIBER ~ 0.2 G TOTAL
FAT ~ 0.0 G SATURATED FAT ~ 0.0 MG CHOLESTEROL ~ 2.0 MG SODIUM

Sprouts are so easy to grow, taste delicious, and offer a large amount of
the enzymes needed to aid in digestion. You can add them to salads, stir-
fries, and many other meals. Since childhood, I have loved to snack on
them raw. My mother taught me how to grow sprouts at a young age,
and I enjoyed tending to them with anticipation. Growing sprouts is a
fun project to teach your children. They will be so excited to eat something they have grown themselves (they forget that sprouts are healthy).
Allow four days for the sprouts to grow.

1/3 cup alfalfa seeds

Filtered water

Special equipment:

Large Mason jar

Cheesecloth

Place the seeds in the jar. Add enough filtered water to cover the seeds.
Cover the top with 2–3 thicknesses of cheesecloth, and secure with a
strong rubber band or with the metal rim that fits the jar.

Place the jar in a warm place away from direct sunlight. Let the
seeds soak for 6–8 hours.

After this initial soaking, rinse the seeds through the cheesecloth.
Drain out excess water. Then turn the jar upside down and place it on a
plate; this allows the water to drain. Rinse 3–4 times per day. Sprouts
should be ready to eat in about 4 days.

Serves 1.

Substitutions

If it is a bean, it will sprout. Even if it is not a bean, it will probably
sprout. The most familiar sprouts are mung bean sprouts and alfalfa
sprouts, but you could
sprout anything and it will
make your salads that much
more exciting. Try radish
seeds, soybeans, cranberry
beans, fava beans, lentils,
barley, rye, oats, chick peas,
mustard seeds, clover seeds,
millet, sunflower seeds—the

Nutritional Analysis per Serving			
Vitamin A	5.3 RE	Vitamin D	0.0 µg
Thiamin (B-1)	0.0 mg	Vitamin E	0.0 mg
Riboflavin (B-2)	0.0 mg	Calcium	10.6 mg
Niacin	0.2 mg	Iron	0.3 mg
Vitamin B-6	0.0 mg	Phosphorus	23.1 mg
Vitamin B-12	0.0 µg	Magnesium	8.9 mg
Folate (total)	11.9 µg	Zinc	0.3 mg
Vitamin C	2.7 mg	Potassium	26.1 mg

list goes on. My favorites are alfalfa seeds mixed with a few radish seeds. Be careful, because the radish seeds are very spicy (I expect mustard seeds are, as well).

Healthy Tidbit

During World War II, when the United States was concerned about a possible meat shortage, the scientific community advised the president that the consumption of germinated seeds was the best and cheapest alternative to proteins in meat. Many sprouts offer a complete protein. In addition they are rich in vitamins, minerals, and natural enzymes. All you need are clean water and 4 days to grow a fully grown, crispy, organic, tasty vegetable. Eat sprouts before a large meal to increase your digestive ability.

Avocado Tuna Salad

PER SERVING: 222.7 CALORIES ~ 30.1 G PROTEIN ~ 4.9 G CARBOHYDRATE ~ 3.8 G FIBER ~ 9.2 G
TOTAL FAT ~ 1.5 G SATURATED FAT ~ 34.0 MG CHOLESTEROL ~ 387.3 MG SODIUM

Try this salad when you want a nutritious, tasty lunch and don't have much time for preparation.

1 ripe medium avocado

2 6-ounce cans of light tuna, in water

½ teaspoon sea salt (optional)

¼–½ teaspoon pepper

Mash avocado. Add tuna and pepper.

Mix together, and serve on rice crackers, salad greens, or nonwheat bread. My favorite is to serve it over lettuce leaves.

Serves 3.

Substitutions

Canned salmon can be used in place of canned tuna. You can add a little cumin, thyme, or dried basil.

Healthy Tidbit

Tuna is a cold-water fish that is high in omega-3 essential fatty acids. Because it can be a source of mercury, tuna should be rotated in the diet. I generally suggest eating tuna no more than two times per month. Heavy metals such as mercury have the potential to bind irreversibly to sites otherwise available for regulatory molecules that assist in cellular function. They can reduce immune function and interfere with regular metabolism.

Nutritional Analysis per Serving			
Vitamin A	53.9 RE	Vitamin D	0.0 µg
Thiamin (B-1)	0.1 mg	Vitamin E	0.8 mg
Riboflavin (B-2)	0.2 mg	Calcium	20.0 mg
Niacin	16.0 mg	Iron	2.1 mg
Vitamin B-6	0.5 mg	Phosphorus	214.6 mg
Vitamin B-12	3.4 µg	Magnesium	47.4 mg
Folate (total)	37.4 µg	Zinc	1.2 mg
Vitamin C	5.7 mg	Potassium	545.8 mg

Beet and Bean Salad

PER SERVING: 215.5 CALORIES ~ 5.4 G PROTEIN ~ 21.4 G CARBOHYDRATE ~ 5.3 G FIBER ~ 13.2 G
TOTAL FAT ~ 1.6 G SATURATED FAT ~ 0.0 MG CHOLESTEROL ~ 58.0 MG SODIUM

This delicious, nutritious salad offers a nice change of pace. When I made it for a holiday dinner it was quickly gobbled down.

For the salad:

¼ cup hazelnuts

3–4 large beets, steamed until tender and peeled

1½ cups green beans, cut into bite size pieces and steamed until tender

1 cup cooked white beans

1 pear, cut into thin slices

1 leek, sliced (mostly the white part)

For the dressing:

2 tablespoons fresh dill or 1 teaspoon dry dill

2 cloves garlic, minced

2 teaspoons mustard, no additives or sugar

2 teaspoons balsamic vinegar

¼ cup extra-virgin olive oil

Cut cooked beets into bite-size pieces and combine in a large bowl with green beans, white beans, pear slices, and leek slices.

Prepare dressing by whisking all ingredients together in a small bowl. Pour over salad, mix well, and store in refrigerator for at least 1 hour before serving.

Roast hazelnuts on a cake pan in the oven until golden, about 6–8 minutes. Remove from oven, allow to cool slightly, chop, and set aside until salad is finished marinating. Sprinkle hazelnuts over salad before serving.

Serves 6.

Nutritional Analysis per Serving			
Vitamin A	22.1 RE	Vitamin D	0.0 µg
Thiamin (B-1)	0.1 mg	Vitamin E	1.3 mg
Riboflavin (B-2)	0.1 mg	Calcium	65.5 mg
Niacin	1.0 mg	Iron	2.5 mg
Vitamin B-6	0.2 mg	Phosphorus	87.1 mg
Vitamin B-12	0.0 µg	Magnesium	51.0 mg
Folate (total)	93.4 µg	Zinc	0.8 mg
Vitamin C	9.2 mg	Potassium	457.1 mg

Substitutions
Canned cannelloni or navy beans can be used, among other beans. Experiment with different vegetables, too. Using canned beans makes the recipe easier, but do not use canned beets, green beans, or other vegetables as they lose their nutritional value during the canning process and often contain additives and salt.

Healthy Tidbit
Nuts are an excellent source of protein. Enjoy them as a snack between meals to stabilize blood sugar, or add them to any meal for a protein boost. Different nuts offer different nutritional benefits, but, generally, they are all high in essential fatty acids, and often high in calcium, selenium, and other trace minerals.

Colorful Coleslaw

PER SERVING: 117.0 CALORIES ~ 1.2 G PROTEIN ~ 13.4 G CARBOHYDRATE ~ 2.6 G FIBER ~ 7.3 G
TOTAL FAT ~ 1.0 G SATURATED FAT ~ 0.0 MG CHOLESTEROL ~ 24.5 MG SODIUM

This simple and sweet coleslaw tastes better than any other I've tried.

2 cups shredded red cabbage	3 tablespoons olive oil or flaxseed oil
2 cups shredded white cabbage	2 tablespoons red wine vinegar
4 cups boiling water	1 tablespoon lemon juice
3 carrots, shredded	1 tablespoon honey
1 apple, shredded	1 teaspoon horseradish (from a jar)
¼ cup raisins (optional; omit if you are diabetic)	¼ teaspoon onion powder
½ onion, chopped (optional)	¼ teaspoon garlic powder
2 tablespoons fresh cilantro	Sea salt or tamari to taste

Combine cabbage and raisins in a large bowl. Pour boiling water over them, cover, and let sit for 5 minutes. Drain.

Whisk together liquid ingredients. Add along with all other ingredients to cabbage mixture. Stir well. Store in the refrigerator for at least 2 hours before serving, to allow flavors to mingle.

Serves 6.

Substitutions

For a coleslaw that is less sweet, leave out the raisins, honey, and apple, or use only half an apple.

Healthy Tidbit

Individuals with thyroid problems should not consume certain raw vegetables that contain goitrogens, substances that may potentiate a goiter. Here is a partial list: brussels sprouts, cauliflower, cabbage, broccoli, spinach, beets, kale, and turnips. These should *not* be eaten raw by anyone suffering from thyroid problems.

Nutritional Analysis per Serving			
Vitamin A	1,141.7 RE	Vitamin D	0.0 µg
Thiamin (B-1)	0.1 mg	Vitamin E	1.1 mg
Riboflavin (B-2)	0.0 mg	Calcium	37.6 mg
Niacin	0.9 mg	Iron	0.6 mg
Vitamin B-6	0.1 mg	Phosphorus	37.0 mg
Vitamin B-12	0.0 µg	Magnesium	14.9 mg
Folate (total)	22.3 µg	Zinc	0.2 mg
Vitamin C	27.3 mg	Potassium	270.4 mg

Cucumber Salad

PER SERVING: 45.0 CALORIES ~ 1.3 G PROTEIN ~ 5.0 G CARBOHYDRATE ~ 1.0 G FIBER ~ 2.6 G
TOTAL FAT ~ 0.3 G SATURATED FAT ~ 0.0 MG CHOLESTEROL ~ 4.6 MG SODIUM

This salad goes well with most meat dishes. For a complete anti-inflammatory Mediterranean feast, serve Barbecued Kafta (see page 128), Nut 'n' Curry Hummus (see page 64), Baba Ghanoush (see page 58), and Cucumber Salad. Your guests will love it.

For the salad:

2 large or 3 small cucumbers, sliced thin

½ medium onion, sliced into very thin rings

For the dressing:

1 tablespoon plus 1 teaspoon rice vinegar

2 teaspoons cold-pressed extra-virgin olive oil

Maple syrup to taste (optional)

Sea salt to taste

Pepper to taste

Prepare salad by slicing cucumbers and onion and tossing together in a large bowl.

In a separate, smaller bowl, whisk together rice vinegar, olive oil, and maple syrup, and pour over cucumbers and onions. Toss together and add sea salt and pepper to taste.

Serve cold or at room temperature. It tastes best if it has had time to marinate in the refrigerator for at least 1 hour before serving.

Serves 4.

Healthy Tidbit
Cucumbers are cooling and thirst quenching and can relieve edema (fluid retention). Use fresh slices of cucumber as eye compresses for a refreshing, relaxing effect. Cucumber flesh is added to facial masks and can help soothe sunburn. Cucumbers can cleanse and purify the blood, thereby helping to restore normal health. They also contain a digestive enzyme, erepsin, that breaks down proteins, cleanses the intestines, and helps defend against parasites.

Nutritional Analysis per Serving			
Vitamin A	33.4 RE	Vitamin D	0.0 µg
Thiamin (B-1)	0.0 mg	Vitamin E	0.3 mg
Riboflavin (B-2)	0.0 mg	Calcium	31.1 mg
Niacin	0.4 mg	Iron	0.4 mg
Vitamin B-6	0.1 mg	Phosphorus	42.4 mg
Vitamin B-12	0.0 µg	Magnesium	21.1 mg
Folate (total)	0.0 µg	Zinc	0.2 mg
Vitamin C	9.8 mg	Potassium	282.3 mg

Curried Quinoa Salad

PER SERVING: 695.2 CALORIES ~ 8.9 G PROTEIN ~ 69.2 G CARBOHYDRATE ~ 7.2 G FIBER ~ 45.5 G
TOTAL FAT ~ 6.1 G SATURATED FAT ~ 0.0 MG CHOLESTEROL ~ 315.7 MG SODIUM

This recipe comes from a patient of mine, Cyndi Stuart. This dish combines two of my favorite flavors, curry and quinoa.

For the dressing:

¼ cup fresh lemon juice
2½ teaspoons curry powder
½ teaspoon allspice
½ teaspoon sea salt
½ teaspoon black pepper
¾ cup olive oil

For the salad:

2 cups cooked quinoa
1 bunch green onions, diced
1 medium red pepper, diced
1 cup raisins (omit if you are diabetic)
½ cup cooked or canned chickpeas (garbanzo beans)

In a small bowl, whisk together all the dressing ingredients except the oil.

Gradually add the oil to the dressing mixture in a thin stream, whisking until all is blended. Set dressing aside.

Fluff the quinoa with a fork. Add the remaining salad ingredients, and mix well.

Add dressing, toss, and chill for at least 2 hours or overnight. The flavors really come together as the salad marinates.

Serves 4.

Healthy Tidbit

It is the berry of the allspice plant, ground into a fine powder, that is used as a seasoning. Allspice is a warming herb used to remedy chills and to ease flatulence. The berries and leaves are also used to perfume cosmetics and to flavor teas.

Nutritional Analysis per Serving			
Vitamin A	189.9 RE	Vitamin D	0.0 µg
Thiamin (B-1)	0.2 mg	Vitamin E	5.4 mg
Riboflavin (B-2)	0.3 mg	Calcium	101.8 mg
Niacin	4.1 mg	Iron	6.3 mg
Vitamin B-6	0.3 mg	Phosphorus	246.1 mg
Vitamin B-12	0.0 µg	Magnesium	112.1 mg
Folate (total)	92.2 µg	Zinc	1.9 mg
Vitamin C	73.5 mg	Potassium	852.3 mg

Curry Chicken Salad

PER SERVING: 412.2 CALORIES ~ 33.5 G PROTEIN ~ 13.0 G CARBOHYDRATE ~ 1.5 G FIBER ~ 24.9 G
TOTAL FAT ~ 2.8 G SATURATED FAT ~ 98.5 MG CHOLESTEROL ~ 530.5 MG SODIUM

After enjoying a curry chicken salad sandwich in the deli of a health-food store, I had to come up with a recipe for it.

1¼ pounds organic chicken breast, baked and cubed

½ cup organic mayonnaise (look for one with all natural ingredients)

½ cup diced celery

½ medium fuji apple, diced

¼–½ cup raisins (omit if you are diabetic)

¼ cup diced onion (optional)

2½ teaspoons curry powder

½ teaspoon turmeric

½ teaspoon salt or to taste

Dash of pepper

6 large lettuce leaves (for serving)

Mix together all ingredients, and allow to sit in refrigerator for at least 30 minutes. Serve on lettuce leaves.
Serves 4.

Substitutions
For a vegetarian version, try cubes of firm baked tofu instead of chicken.

Healthy Tidbit
Curry powder, a blend of traditional Indian spices, is one of my favorite seasonings because it is so versatile. It is terrific for egg dishes, meat dishes, salads, and grains. Begin experimenting with curry powder; you can never go wrong.

Nutritional Analysis per Serving			
Vitamin A	29.6 RE	Vitamin D	0.1 µg
Thiamin (B-1)	0.1 mg	Vitamin E	1.4 mg
Riboflavin (B-2)	0.2 mg	Calcium	34.3 mg
Niacin	16.1 mg	Iron	1.6 mg
Vitamin B-6	0.8 mg	Phosphorus	32.6 mg
Vitamin B-12	0.6 µg	Magnesium	52.4 mg
Folate (total)	32.6 µg	Zinc	1.3 mg
Vitamin C	5.4 mg	Potassium	623.3 mg

Curry Garbanzo Salad

PER SERVING: 172.8 CALORIES ~ 12.1 G PROTEIN ~ 35.8 G CARBOHYDRATE ~ 9.1 G FIBER ~ 4.2 G
TOTAL FAT ~ 0.3 G SATURATED FAT ~ 0.0 MG CHOLESTEROL ~ 770.7 MG SODIUM

Here's yet another recipe using the highly adaptable flavor of curry.

For the salad:

2 15-ounce cans of garbanzo beans, drained

½ medium onion, minced

2 stalks celery, diced small

For the dressing:

1 tablespoon plus 1 teaspoon tarragon vinegar

2 teaspoons olive oil

Juice of 1 medium lemon

2 cloves garlic, minced

1 teaspoon curry powder

½ teaspoon cumin

½ teaspoon turmeric

Sea salt to taste

Pepper to taste

In a small bowl, whisk together dressing ingredients. In a larger bowl, toss all ingredients together. Before serving, allow to chill in the refrigerator for 1 or 2 hours or overnight.

Serves 4.

Substitutions

Use less onion and less garlic if you want a milder flavor. For more heat, you can add a small spicy pepper (e.g., a Thai or serrano pepper), minced. Try different vegetables or legumes (e.g., lentils, black beans). Adding roasted red peppers or sundried tomatoes, if tolerable, is a fun, artistic touch that imparts wonderful flavor.

Healthy Tidbit

Cumin is an ancient Mediterranean seasoning that is used in many different cuisines, including Indian, Greek, Mexican, and others. It has a distinctive flavor; therefore you do not need to use a lot. Cumin is a stimulant, a digestive tonic, and a carminative, which means it helps to relieve gas, or flatus.

Nutritional Analysis per Serving			
Vitamin A	3.7 RE	Vitamin D	0.0 µg
Thiamin (B-1)	0.0 mg	Vitamin E	0.3 mg
Riboflavin (B-2)	0.0 mg	Calcium	55.0 mg
Niacin	0.3 mg	Iron	2.2 mg
Vitamin B-6	0.1 mg	Phosphorus	17.3 mg
Vitamin B-12	0.0 µg	Magnesium	7.5 mg
Folate (total)	10.1 µg	Zinc	0.1 mg
Vitamin C	11.6 mg	Potassium	128.4 mg

Garlic Bean Salad

PER SERVING: 101.1 CALORIES ~ 2.2 G PROTEIN ~ 8.8 G CARBOHYDRATE ~ 3.9 G FIBER ~ 7.2 G
TOTAL FAT ~ 1.0 G SATURATED FAT ~ 0.0 MG CHOLESTEROL ~ 7.3 MG SODIUM

Here is another great recipe from acupuncturist Dawn Berry, L.Ac.

1 pound green beans, blanched and cooled

2 tablespoons olive oil

2 teaspoons apple cider vinegar

½ teaspoon thyme

1 garlic clove, minced

1 small shallot, minced

Sea salt and pepper to taste

Prepare the beans by blanching in steam for 2–3 minutes until they are bright green. Set aside to cool.

Whisk together remaining ingredients, and toss with cooled green beans. Place in refrigerator to marinate for 1 hour before serving.

Serves 4.

Healthy Tidbit

Garlic is delectable roasted in the oven and used as a spread. Because of its healing and antimicrobial properties, I make sure to include it in my daily diet. When I have a cold, I make a drink combining 1 minced garlic clove with a small amount of lemon juice, maple syrup, and filtered water. I drink it morning and evening.

Nutritional Analysis per Serving			
Vitamin A	81.7 RE	Vitamin D	0.0 µg
Thiamin (B-1)	0.1 mg	Vitamin E	0.8 mg
Riboflavin (B-2)	0.1 mg	Calcium	46.1 mg
Niacin	1.1 mg	Iron	1.5 mg
Vitamin B-6	0.1 mg	Phosphorus	41.2 mg
Vitamin B-12	0.0 µg	Magnesium	28.3 mg
Folate (total)	28.0 µg	Zinc	0.3 mg
Vitamin C	14.3 mg	Potassium	223.9 mg

Italian Carrot Salad

PER SERVING: 116.4 CALORIES ~ 1.4 G PROTEIN ~ 12.5 G CARBOHYDRATE ~ 3.0 G FIBER ~ 7.3 G
TOTAL FAT ~ 1.0 G SATURATED FAT ~ 0.0 MG CHOLESTEROL ~ 40.8 MG SODIUM

I learned how to make this salad when I lived with an Italian family during college. It complements any dinner or tastes great as a midafternoon snack.

1 pound carrots, cut into 3-inch-long, thin sticks

2 tablespoons red wine vinegar

2 tablespoons olive oil

1 teaspoon dried basil

3 garlic cloves, minced fine or pressed

Sea salt to taste (optional)

Pepper to taste

Steam the carrot sticks till crisp-tender.

In a small bowl, whisk together remaining ingredients.

Toss together carrots and dressing in a sealable container. Allow carrots to cool, seal container, and invert a few times.

Store in refrigerator until serving time (at least 1 hour, prefereably overnight). Periodically invert the container.

Serves 4.

Healthy Tidbit

Olive oil is a monounsaturated fat that can promote healthy lipid profiles in the body. It helps to decrease the "bad" cholesterol, or LDL cholesterol, and increase the "good" cholesterol, HDL cholesterol. Because olive oil is unsaturated and contains a double bond, it is easily broken down by the body and incorporated into important hormones and cell membranes.

Nutritional Analysis per Serving			
Vitamin A	2,885.0 RE	Vitamin D	0.0 µg
Thiamin (B-1)	0.1 mg	Vitamin E	1.4 mg
Riboflavin (B-2)	0.1 mg	Calcium	43.2 mg
Niacin	1.4 mg	Iron	0.8 mg
Vitamin B-6	0.2 mg	Phosphorus	55.2 mg
Vitamin B-12	0.0 µg	Magnesium	19.1 mg
Folate (total)	13.8 µg	Zinc	0.3 mg
Vitamin C	8.9 mg	Potassium	388.7 mg

Mexican Salad

PER SERVING: 103.6 CALORIES ~ 6.2 G PROTEIN ~ 18.9 G CARBOHYDRATE ~ 6.5 G FIBER ~ 2.3 G
TOTAL FAT ~ 0.3 G SATURATED FAT ~ 0.0 MG CHOLESTEROL ~ 470.6 MG SODIUM

I prepare this dressing often to top salads or fish. Try it with this salad
and with others; it will become a favorite.

For the salad:

1 head of red leaf or green leaf lettuce,
shredded

1 small bunch of red radishes, grated

2 tablespoons minced cilantro

1 15-ounce can cooked black beans,
drained

For the dressing:

3 tablespoons fresh lemon juice

3 tablespoons tahini

1 tablespoon apple cider vinegar

2 teaspoons mustard (make sure it does
not have any ingredients excluded in the
anti-inflammatory diet)

4 tablespoons filtered water

Combine lettuce leaves, radishes, and cilantro. Pour beans over the top.
In a small bowl or large cup, whisk together dressing ingredients.
Drizzle dressing over salad, and serve. Serves 4.

Substitutions

There are many ways to modify this salad. You can use tarragon vinegar
instead of apple cider vinegar. One of my favorite variations is to bake
salmon, season it with a little lemon, and place it on top of the beans
before adding the dressing. You may need to make a little more dressing
if you are adding salmon. Also try adding tomatoes, if tolerated, or avocados.

Healthy Tidbit

Apple cider vinegar is helpful as a digestive stimulant if taken before a
meal. Stir 1–2 teaspoons vinegar into 4–8 fluid ounces of water and
drink it 15 minutes before eating. It will help to increase production of
stomach acid for the breakdown of food. Apple cider vinegar contains a
cholesterol-reducing pectin
and many minerals, including potassium, phosphorus,
chlorine, sodium, magne-
sium, calcium, sulfur, iron,
fluorine, and silicon. It has
been used for centuries to
treat various conditions
and to aid in weight loss.

Nutritional Analysis per Serving			
Vitamin A	0.5 RE	Vitamin D	0.0 µg
Thiamin (B-1)	0.1 mg	Vitamin E	0.2 mg
Riboflavin (B-2)	0.1 mg	Calcium	96.2 mg
Niacin	0.5 mg	Iron	2.8 mg
Vitamin B-6	0.1 mg	Phosphorus	53.7 mg
Vitamin B-12	0.0 µg	Magnesium	14.8 mg
Folate (total)	33.0 µg	Zinc	0.3 mg
Vitamin C	16.1 mg	Potassium	547.2 mg

Quinoa Vegetable Salad

PER SERVING: 284.0 CALORIES ~ 20.8 G PROTEIN ~ 31.0 G CARBOHYDRATE ~ 3.7 G FIBER ~ 9.4 G TOTAL FAT ~ 1.0 G SATURATED FAT ~ 46.7 MG CHOLESTEROL ~ 84.7 MG SODIUM

It seems that no matter how I change this salad it always turns out good. Amazingly, it contains no spices.

2 cups leftover cooked boneless, skinless chicken, cubed

1 cup cooked quinoa, or $^1/_3$ cup dried quinoa

1 medium apple, peeled and chopped

2 stalks celery, chopped

1 medium carrot, shredded

¼ cup walnuts

$^1/_3$ cup raisins (omit if you are diabetic)

1½ tablespoons organic mayonnaise (with no preservatives or hydrogenated oils)

4 large lettuce leaves (for serving)

Cook quinoa according to the directions on page 166, or use leftover quinoa.

Toss all ingredients together, and serve chilled over lettuce leaves. Serves 4.

Substitutions
You could substitute many different kinds of chopped fruits, nuts, or raw vegetables. You could use canned salmon or leftover turkey in place of the chicken. This salad is even great if you leave out the meat completely.

Healthy Tidbit
Quinoa is a high-energy grain that is easy to digest. Unlike many other grains, quinoa contains complete protein, meaning it has each of the essential amino acids. It contains more calcium than milk, equals milk's protein content, and is high in the amino acid lysine. Include quinoa in your diet often if you suffer from outbreaks of cold sores.

Nutritional Analysis per Serving			
Vitamin A	585.5 RE	Vitamin D	0.0 µg
Thiamin (B-1)	0.1 mg	Vitamin E	0.8 mg
Riboflavin (B-2)	0.2 mg	Calcium	42.2 mg
Niacin	5.7 mg	Iron	2.6 mg
Vitamin B-6	0.3 mg	Phosphorus	132.0 mg
Vitamin B-12	0.1 µg	Magnesium	72.7 mg
Folate (total)	35.1 µg	Zinc	1.4 mg
Vitamin C	5.3 mg	Potassium	603.7 mg

Carrot Beet Salad

PER SERVING: 156.1 CALORIES ~ 2.1 G PROTEIN ~ 13.0 G CARBOHYDRATE ~ 2.7 G FIBER ~ 11.4 G
TOTAL FAT ~ 1.6 G SATURATED FAT ~ 0.0 MG CHOLESTEROL ~ 329.8 MG SODIUM

My good friend and colleague Wendy Abraham, N.D., inspired this
salad.

For the dressing:

4 tablespoons apple cider vinegar

3 tablespoons olive oil

2 tablespoons mustard (select one containing no additives or sugar)

¼ teaspoon sea salt or to taste

¼ teaspoon pepper or to taste

For the salad:

½ pound carrots, grated

3 raw beets, peeled and grated

Mix dressing ingredients together; taste, and adjust seasonings as you
desire. Add grated beets and grated carrots; toss to coat with dressing.
Serve chilled.
Serves 4.

Substitutions
You could try different salad dressings. You could also add a few grated
radishes for a hint of spice.

Healthy Tidbit
Beets are a blood tonic, which makes them great for treating anemia,
heart conditions, and circulation. Beet greens are high in many nutrients,
including calcium, magnesium, iron, phosphorus, and vitamins pro-A, B-
complex, and C. Be sure to save your beet greens for the next night's
stir-fry.

Nutritional Analysis per Serving			
Vitamin A	1,443.3 RE	Vitamin D	0.0 µg
Thiamin (B-1)	0.1 mg	Vitamin E	2.1 mg
Riboflavin (B-2)	0.1 mg	Calcium	39.2 mg
Niacin	1.2 mg	Iron	1.2 mg
Vitamin B-6	0.1 mg	Phosphorus	63.0 mg
Vitamin B-12	0.0 µg	Magnesium	27.7 mg
Folate (total)	73.3 µg	Zinc	0.4 mg
Vitamin C	7.0 mg	Potassium	410.2 mg

Spicy Honey Lemon Salad

PER SERVING: 145.2 CALORIES ~ 1.1 G PROTEIN ~ 39.4 G CARBOHYDRATE ~ 1.0 G FIBER ~ 0.1 G
TOTAL FAT ~ 0.0 G SATURATED FAT ~ 0.0 MG CHOLESTEROL ~ 607.2 MG SODIUM

The dressing included with this salad is quick and easy when you want
something tasty to go on any tossed greens.

²/₃ cup lemon juice (juice of about 3–4 lemons)

½ cup honey

2 teaspoons grated lemon zest

1 teaspoon sea salt

Generous pinch of cayenne pepper

4 cups of fresh spinach

Mix together all dressing ingredients in a small bowl. Pour mixture over
spinach greens and toss gently.

Serves 4.

Substitutions

I like to add grated radishes to my salad for extra zing. They complement the spice of the cayenne pepper in this dressing very well. If you
want a thicker dressing, make it slightly ahead of time and refrigerate for
a while, or add 1–2 tablespoons tahini and mix well.

Healthy Tidbit

Eating a salad before a meal is not just a custom that we have adopted
by accident. Eating salad greens offers the body a bitter flavor, which
stimulates the production of digestive enzymes and stomach acid. In
addition, the acidic lemon or vinegar in salad dressings also stimulates
digestion to begin. If you are given the choice, always choose to enjoy
your salad before your main course.

Nutritional Analysis per Serving			
Vitamin A	202.5 RE	Vitamin D	0.0 µg
Thiamin (B-1)	0.0 mg	Vitamin E	0.0 mg
Riboflavin (B-2)	0.1 mg	Calcium	36.8 mg
Niacin	0.3 mg	Iron	1.0 mg
Vitamin B-6	0.1 mg	Phosphorus	18.9 mg
Vitamin B-12	0.0 µg	Magnesium	27.1 mg
Folate (total)	64.4 µg	Zinc	0.3 mg
Vitamin C	28.6 mg	Potassium	241.4 mg

Spicy Raspberry Vinaigrette Salad

PER SERVING: 48.6 CALORIES ~ 1.2 G PROTEIN ~ 3.5 G CARBOHYDRATE ~ 1.4 G FIBER ~ 3.6 G
TOTAL FAT ~ 2.9 G SATURATED FAT ~ 0.0 MG CHOLESTEROL ~ 19.3 MG SODIUM

This delicious dressing comes from Myra Wilbur of McMinnville, Oregon, who has been very creative about experimenting with the anti-inflammation diet.

For the dressing:

½ cup raspberries

¼ cup red wine vinegar

1 tablespoon coconut oil, warmed to a liquid consistency

Lots of black pepper

For the salad:

1 head of red leaf or green leaf lettuce, or a large bunch of mixed greens

Prepare dressing by blending all ingredients together in the blender.
Pour dressing over top of the greens and serve immediately.
Serves 4.

Substitutions

As with any salad, you can pretty much add anything and it will taste great if the dressing is good. You can use olive oil or flaxseed oil in place of coconut oil. You can use different berries, such as organic strawberries.

Healthy Tidbit

Raspberries are very easy to grow in many different climates. Tea from the leaves can be used in the last trimester of pregnancy to tone the uterine and pelvic muscles to prepare them for labor.

Nutritional Analysis per Serving			
Vitamin A	2.0 RE	Vitamin D	0.0 µg
Thiamin (B-1)	0.1 mg	Vitamin E	0.1 mg
Riboflavin (B-2)	0.1 mg	Calcium	28.9 mg
Niacin	0.4 mg	Iron	1.0 mg
Vitamin B-6	0.1 mg	Phosphorus	23.5 mg
Vitamin B-12	0.0 µg	Magnesium	12.0 mg
Folate (total)	31.8 µg	Zinc	0.2 mg
Vitamin C	6.7 mg	Potassium	167.8 mg

Strawberry Spinach Salad

PER SERVING: 465.2 CALORIES ~ 5.9 G PROTEIN ~ 34.1 G CARBOHYDRATE ~ 6.7 G FIBER ~ 36.2 G
TOTAL FAT ~ 4.6 G SATURATED FAT ~ 0.0 MG CHOLESTEROL ~ 66.8 MG SODIUM

I found a version of this recipe on the Internet, which is a good resource for recipes once you are comfortable substituting ingredients to make the dish conform to the anti-inflammatory diet.

For the dressing:
2 tablespoons sesame seeds
1 tablespoon poppy seeds
½ cup olive oil
¼ cup honey
¼ cup red wine vinegar
¼ teaspoon paprika
¼ teaspoon mustard
1 tablespoon dried minced onion

For the salad:
10-ounce bag fresh spinach leaves, chopped, washed, and dried
1 quart organic strawberries, sliced
¼ cup toasted, slivered almonds

Whisk together dressing ingredients.

In a large bowl, combine spinach, strawberries, and almonds.

Pour dressing over salad, toss, and refrigerate 10–15 minutes before serving.

Serves 4.

Substitutions
Try this salad with avocados, other nuts (e.g., cashews, walnuts, hazelnuts), and fruits (e.g., blueberries, diced pear).

Healthy Tidbit
Many of us do not eat enough green leafy vegetables. They offer many nutrients, including calcium and lutein, which is a powerful antioxidant for eye health. Lutein has been proven helpful in preventing macular degeneration.

Nutritional Analysis per Serving			
Vitamin A	489.3 RE	Vitamin D	0.0 µg
Thiamin (B-1)	0.2 mg	Vitamin E	5.7 mg
Riboflavin (B-2)	0.3 mg	Calcium	193.0 mg
Niacin	2.8 mg	Iron	4.1 mg
Vitamin B-6	0.3 mg	Phosphorus	153.8 mg
Vitamin B-12	0.0 µg	Magnesium	121.7 mg
Folate (total)	171.2 µg	Zinc	1.5 mg
Vitamin C	102.7 mg	Potassium	758.6 mg

Tasty Lemon Vinaigrette Salad

PER SERVING: 294.7 CALORIES ~ 3.5 G PROTEIN ~ 9.9 G CARBOHYDRATE ~ 1.6 G FIBER ~ 28.2 G
TOTAL FAT ~ 3.0 G SATURATED FAT ~ 0.0 MG CHOLESTEROL ~ 426.4 MG SODIUM

This was my basic dressing for years before I ventured to experiment further. It tastes good, it's easy, and I always have the ingredients to make it in a pinch.

For the dressing:

¼ cup lemon juice

¼ cup olive oil or flaxseed oil

2 tablespoons balsamic vinegar

1 tablespoon pure maple syrup

½ teaspoon red pepper flakes

1 teaspoon dried basil

For the salad:

1 head of red leaf or green leaf lettuce

½ cup kalamata olives, pitted and whole

½ cup pine nuts

In a small skillet over medium heat, toast pine nuts in a small amount of oil until golden brown. Toss with lettuce leaves and olives.

In a separate bowl, mix dressing. Pour over top of salad.

Serves 4.

Substitutions

Flaxseed oil is always a healthy substitute for olive oil in salads. And besides experimenting with different types of fruits and nuts, you can try adding grated raw carrots, radishes, or beets.

Healthy Tidbit

The olive tree is a long-lived, drought-resistant evergreen. That's what makes olives an excellent oil-yielding fruit. Besides olive oil, which is high in antioxidants, the olive leaf has antiviral properties. I have found olive leaf extract to be very helpful in treating herpes outbreaks and chronic sinusitis.

Nutritional Analysis per Serving

Vitamin A	18.7 RE	Vitamin D	0.0 µg
Thiamin (B-1)	0.1 mg	Vitamin E	2.2 mg
Riboflavin (B-2)	0.1 mg	Calcium	52.7 mg
Niacin	1.8 mg	Iron	2.5 mg
Vitamin B-6	0.1 mg	Phosphorus	126.5 mg
Vitamin B-12	0.0 µg	Magnesium	55.9 mg
Folate (total)	36.8 µg	Zinc	1.5 mg
Vitamin C	10.4 mg	Potassium	301.6 mg

The Not-So-Greek Salad

PER SERVING: 357.4 CALORIES ~ 2.5 G PROTEIN ~ 7.8 G CARBOHYDRATE ~ 2.1 G FIBER ~ 36.5 G
TOTAL FAT ~ 4.5 G SATURATED FAT ~ 0.0 MG CHOLESTEROL ~ 994.8 MG SODIUM

But Greek enough to make it a fine accompaniment to your Mediterranean feast of kafta, hummus, and baba ghanoush.

For the dressing:	*For the salad:*
½ cup cold-pressed olive oil	1 head romaine lettuce, chopped
½ cup fresh-squeezed lemon juice	1 cup thinly sliced cucumbers
4 cloves garlic, minced	½ cup kalamata olives, pitted and whole
1 teaspoon dried oregano	¼ cup pine nuts
1 teaspoon black pepper	
1 teaspoon salt	

In a small skillet over medium heat, toast pine nuts in a small amount of oil till golden brown.

Prepare salad by tossing greens with cucumbers, olives, and pine nuts. In a small bowl combine all dressing ingredients and mix well. Pour over salad and serve immediately.

Serves 4.

Substitutions
You can add other favorite salad toppers, such as grated raw carrots, fresh tomatoes (if tolerable), chopped red or green bell pepper, or sliced pepperoncinis.

Healthy Tidbit
Garlic was used by the ancient Greeks for more than just feeding their bellies. They would set it atop cairns at crossroads to propitiate Hecate, the underworld goddess of magic, charms, and enchantment. Garlic has many healing properties. It is antimicrobial, antiseptic, antifungal, antiparasitic, and has anticancer effects. It is warming, stimulating, and helps to stabilize blood sugar levels. Garlic helps thin the blood, thereby reducing cardiovascular risk. These are only a few of garlic's magical powers; I suggest you experiment with it often in your cooking.

Nutritional Analysis per Serving			
Vitamin A	160.4 RE	Vitamin D	0.0 µg
Thiamin (B-1)	0.1 mg	Vitamin E	3.9 mg
Riboflavin (B-2)	0.1 mg	Calcium	55.1 mg
Niacin	2.1 mg	Iron	2.1 mg
Vitamin B-6	0.1 mg	Phosphorus	83.4 mg
Vitamin B-12	0.0 µg	Magnesium	37.5 mg
Folate (total)	84.2 µg	Zinc	0.8 mg
Vitamin C	30.3 mg	Potassium	307.3 mg

Soups

Dr. Jason's Savory Mushroom Soup

PER SERVING: 191.6 CALORIES ~ 5.0 G PROTEIN ~ 27.7 G CARBOHYDRATE ~ 5.7 G FIBER ~ 8.4 G
TOTAL FAT ~ 1.1 G SATURATED FAT ~ 0.0 MG CHOLESTEROL ~ 714.3 MG SODIUM

This recipe was developed by my husband, Jason Black, N.D. It affords wonderful immune-boosting properties.

3 tablespoons olive oil	2 cups sliced shiitake mushrooms
2 medium onions, chopped	2 cups sliced crimini mushrooms
4 celery stalks, chopped	7 cups organic chicken broth
6 garlic cloves, minced or pressed	3 tablespoons yellow miso paste
1 tablespoon dried rosemary	3 bay leaves
1 tablespoon dried sage	Sea salt to taste
1 tablespoon dried thyme	Black pepper to taste
4 large carrots, chopped	

Sauté onions, celery, garlic, rosemary, sage, and thyme over medium heat in a large soup pot until onions and celery are translucent.

Add carrots and mushrooms and sauté for another 3 minutes.

Add broth, miso paste, and bay leaves, reduce heat, and simmer for 20–30 minutes.

Taste, and add sea salt and pepper as desired.

Serves 6.

Healthy Tidbit

According to an article published in 2003 in the journal *Life Science* that reviewed a study performed at the Chinese University of Hong Kong, lentin, a protein found in shiitake mushrooms, acts as a strong antifungal and has been shown to decrease the proliferation of leukemia cells. It also revealed inhibitory action against HIV-reverse transcriptase, which could prove effective in preventing HIV patients from developing AIDS.

Nutritional Analysis per Serving			
Vitamin A	1,667.4 RE	Vitamin D	0.0 µg
Thiamin (B-1)	0.1 mg	Vitamin E	1.2 mg
Riboflavin (B-2)	0.2 mg	Calcium	99.7 mg
Niacin	1.9 mg	Iron	2.7 mg
Vitamin B-6	0.3 mg	Phosphorus	360.2 mg
Vitamin B-12	0.0 µg	Magnesium	30.4 mg
Folate (total)	33.6 µg	Zinc	1.1 mg
Vitamin C	11.5 mg	Potassium	703.7 mg

Winter Soup

PER SERVING: 262.5 CALORIES ~ 6.9 G PROTEIN ~ 39.5 G CARBOHYDRATE ~ 7.8 G FIBER ~ 9.7 G
TOTAL FAT ~ 1.3 G SATURATED FAT ~ 0.0 MG CHOLESTEROL ~ 1,600.6 MG SODIUM

This recipe was given to me by my friend and colleague Matt Fisel, N.D. He could always be counted on to bring the most creative dishes to potlucks.

½ medium butternut squash, peeled and cubed

4 medium carrots, sliced

⅓ cup sliced burdock root, found in the bulk herb section of most health-food stores

¼ cup chopped turmeric root or ½ teaspoon turmeric powder, found in the bulk herb section of most health-food stores

2 tablespoons olive oil

½ medium onion, chopped

4 tablespoons grated fresh ginger

8 cloves garlic, chopped

8 cups vegetable stock

2 tablespoons fresh parsley, chopped

1 teaspoon cayenne pepper

1 teaspoon curry powder

Salt to taste

3 lemon slices

4 whole leaves of kale, roughly chopped

¼ cup miso paste

¼ cup sliced green onions (for garnish)

In a large soup pot, sauté the squash, carrots, burdock, and turmeric root in oil on medium-high heat for 5–10 minutes or until ingredients are tender. If using tumeric powder instead of the root, wait to add it until adding the other dry spices.

Add the onions, ginger, and garlic, and cook 5 minutes more. Pour in the stock, and add the parsley, cayenne, curry, salt, lemon slices, and kale; simmer on medium-low heat for 40 minutes.

Remove from heat, stir in miso, and let stand 5 minutes before garnishing with green onions and serving.

Serves 4.

Substitutions

If you have some ingredients but lack others, make substitutions. Use water or organic chicken broth if you don't have vegetable broth. Do, however, try to include garlic, onions, and burdock root, which are all

Nutritional Analysis per Serving			
Vitamin A	3,124.3 RE	Vitamin D	0.0 µg
Thiamin (B-1)	0.2 mg	Vitamin E	1.3 mg
Riboflavin (B-2)	0.1 mg	Calcium	145.4 mg
Niacin	2.4 mg	Iron	2.9 mg
Vitamin B-6	0.4 mg	Phosphorus	769.1 mg
Vitamin B-12	0.0 µg	Magnesium	60.6 mg
Folate (total)	43.8 µg	Zinc	1.0 mg
Vitamin C	41.8 mg	Potassium	1,221.2 mg

healing vegetables that will strengthen your immune system through the cold months.

Healthy Tidbit

Burdock root supports the liver, gallbladder, kidneys, and skin, and helps to sooth mucous membranes. It can act as an alterative (any herb or substance that improves lymphatic circulation, cleanses blood, boosts immunity, and helps to gradually treat chronic conditions), is antibacterial and antifungal, and can be used as a mild diuretic. Because of its bitter properties, it can act as a great digestive stimulant. It is contraindicated in pregnancy.

Clean-Out-the-Refrigerator Soup

PER SERVING: 341.7 CALORIES ~ 26.6 G PROTEIN ~ 46.5 G CARBOHYDRATE ~ 10.2 G FIBER ~ 5.7 G
TOTAL FAT ~ 1.3 G SATURATED FAT ~ 36.3 MG CHOLESTEROL ~ 742.0 MG SODIUM

This is the best way to get rid of those extra vegetables in your crisper
drawer. It is easy for soups to end up tasting the same. Following the
steps outlined here, you can make many different-tasting soups that are
always a hit. The recipe is very versatile because how it turns out really
depends on what you have in your refrigerator.

All of the ingredients listed below are optional; they are merely suggestions to get you started.

For the broth:

6 cups organic chicken stock

1 onion, minced

3 garlic cloves, minced or pressed

2 tablespoons garlic bean sauce (from Asian section of supermarket)

2 tablespoons miso soup paste

Herbs, spices, and sea salt to taste

Additional ingredients:

½ cup oats, ground in a coffee grinder or blender (for a thickener)

½ cup lentils, soaked overnight and water discarded

3 large carrots, sliced

3 celery stalks, sliced

1 large zucchini, sliced

10 shiitake mushrooms, sliced

1 medium sweet potato, cubed

2 cups leftover boneless, skinless chicken

The key to a good-tasting soup is to get the broth right before adding
vegetables and/or meat. Before turning on the stove, taste the broth cold
and adjust the seasonings.
Start by combining chicken
stock with onions and garlic in a soup pot.

Add herbs, spices, gar-
lic bean sauce, miso, or
anything else you desire.
When the taste meets your
satisfaction, turn the

Nutritional Analysis per Serving

Vitamin A	1,588.8 RE	Vitamin D	2.5 µg
Thiamin (B-1)	0.5 mg	Vitamin E	0.3 mg
Riboflavin (B-2)	0.5 mg	Calcium	71.6 mg
Niacin	9.2 mg	Iron	3.5 mg
Vitamin B-6	0.7 mg	Phosphorus	288.1 mg
Vitamin B-12	0.1 µg	Magnesium	94.3 mg
Folate (total)	132.7 µg	Zinc	2.9 mg
Vitamin C	14.3 mg	Potassium	1,061.0 mg

burner to medium high, bring the broth to a boil, then immediately reduce heat and simmer for 15 minutes, covered. Keep tasting and adding seasonings as desired.

For a thicker broth, you can add ground oats at this time. Also add legumes. Don't use too many of these ingredients, because they are dense. Simmer, covered, for another 15 minutes.

Add vegetables, and simmer, covered, for another 15 minutes. Add leftover meat and simmer, covered, for another 15–30 minutes.

After the vegetables have cooked to your satisfaction, turn off the heat and allow the soup to sit covered for at least 15 minutes before serving; this step allows the flavors to mingle. Serve plain or with rice crackers.

Serves 6.

Substitutions

As I've said, you can and should try anything in this soup. Season the broth with tamari instead of or in addition to garlic bean sauce. Add a pinch of dried herbs such as thyme, marjoram, or Herbes de Provence. Use ground quinoa as a thickener instead of oats. Use split peas, barley, or navy beans instead of lentils. Use leftover meat of any kind, including turkey or fish.

Healthy Tidbit

Celery is a great blood cleanser and helps to reduce blood pressure. It helps to remove liver congestion and can ease constipation. It has been used to treat rheumatism, gout, and arthritis. It is fairly dense with water and contains very few calories; therefore, snack on it often.

Cream of Carrot and Ginger Soup

PER SERVING: 289.9 CALORIES ~ 4.8 G PROTEIN ~ 25.0 G CARBOHYDRATE ~ 5.2 G FIBER ~ 19.8 G
TOTAL FAT ~ 11.3 G SATURATED FAT ~ 0.0 MG CHOLESTEROL ~ 418.1 MG SODIUM

If you didn't know, you wouldn't guess that this soup contains no dairy.
It is so creamy that it can satisfy those urges you sometimes get when
dairy is not an option. This is a favorite for all ages.

2 pounds organic carrots

6 garlic cloves

2 medium yellow onions

2 tablespoons olive oil

2 cups organic chicken broth

1 ⅓ cups coconut milk

⅓ cup soy milk

2 teaspoons grated fresh ginger

½ teaspoon sea salt

½ teaspoon pepper

2 tablespoons dried parsley (as garnish)

Steam the carrots until soft.

While the carrots are steaming, sauté the garlic and onions in the
olive oil until they are softened and slightly brown in color.

Combine steamed carrots, cooked garlic and onions, and all remaining ingredients in a blender. Blend on the purée setting. (*Caution: Don't
heat the liquid ingredients before blending*. Using a blender to mix large
quantities of hot liquids can cause a rapid expansion in the liquids,
which can create a small explosion! If you have to blend hot liquids in a
blender, do so in several small batches.)

Heat the blended soup in a large saucepan, and serve garnished with
dried parsley. Serves 6.

Substitutions

Rice milk or almond milk
can be used in place of the
soy milk. To reduce fat,
substitute soy milk, rice
milk, or water for the
coconut milk. To make a
thinner soup, add filtered
water.

Nutritional Analysis per Serving			
Vitamin A	4,319.3 RE	Vitamin D	0.0 µg
Thiamin (B-1)	0.2 mg	Vitamin E	1.8 mg
Riboflavin (B-2)	0.1 mg	Calcium	83.6 mg
Niacin	2.1 mg	Iron	2.3 mg
Vitamin B-6	0.3 mg	Phosphorus	233.8 mg
Vitamin B-12	0.0 µg	Magnesium	53.1 mg
Folate (total)	32.5 µg	Zinc	0.8 mg
Vitamin C	19.3 mg	Potassium	913.2 mg

Healthy Tidbit

Carrots are high in the powerful antioxidants known as carotenoids, which are a vitamin A precursor (that is, they form vitamin A once in the body). Vitamin A is naturally antiviral. Carrots help to support the lungs, liver, pancreas, and kidneys. They improve night vision, skin health, and are anticarcinogenic.

Dr. Fisel's Squash Soup

PER SERVING: 172.1 CALORIES ~ 2.8 G PROTEIN ~ 32.7 G CARBOHYDRATE ~ 5.2 G FIBER ~ 4.1 G
TOTAL FAT ~ 0.6 G SATURATED FAT ~ 0.0 MG CHOLESTEROL ~ 562.5 MG SODIUM

I remember many cold days when Matt Fisel, N.D., would aromatize the medical school lounge with his scrumptious-smelling squash soup. We all would stand in line for a sample.

1 medium onion, chopped

1 tablespoon olive oil

2 cups vegetable stock

2 cups butternut squash (seeds removed), peeled and diced

2 cups sweet potatoes or yams, peeled and diced

1 apple, cored and diced

1 teaspoon freshly grated ginger

½ teaspoon nutmeg

½ teaspoon salt

½ teaspoon pepper

¼ teaspoon cayenne pepper

In a large soup pot, sauté the onions in oil on medium-high heat until translucent.

Add all other ingredients and bring to a boil.

Turn down heat and simmer for 30 minutes.

Remove 2 ladles of vegetables and 1 ladle of stock; purée them together in a blender or food processor until smooth. Return to soup pot; stir soup before serving.

Serves 4.

Healthy Tidbit

Nutmeg is a seed from a fragrant evergreen. The seeds can be roasted, ground, and applied to wounds. Crushed seeds yield a beneficial insecticide. The root can be chewed to relieve a toothache.

Nutritional Analysis per Serving			
Vitamin A	1,935.7 RE	Vitamin D	0.0 µg
Thiamin (B-1)	0.1 mg	Vitamin E	0.5 mg
Riboflavin (B-2)	0.1 mg	Calcium	77.5 mg
Niacin	1.5 mg	Iron	1.3 mg
Vitamin B-6	0.3 mg	Phosphorus	235.6 mg
Vitamin B-12	0.0 µg	Magnesium	47.8 mg
Folate (total)	27.4 µg	Zinc	0.4 mg
Vitamin C	20.8 mg	Potassium	700.4 mg

Nutty Onion Soup

PER SERVING: 543.1 CALORIES ~ 12.5 G PROTEIN ~ 33.9 G CARBOHYDRATE ~ 4.4 G FIBER ~ 43.1 G
TOTAL FAT ~ 7.7 G SATURATED FAT ~ 0.0 MG CHOLESTEROL ~ 475.1 MG SODIUM

This recipe was inspired by another of my favorite cookbooks, Jane Kinderlehrer's *Confessions of a Sneaky Organic Cook*. My daughter chows down on this soup each time I make it. Notice that it has no added salt and really doesn't need any.

1 quart of organic chicken broth

1½ cups filtered water

2 cups cashews

2 small onions, chopped

3 tablespoons cold-pressed, extra-virgin olive oil

2 teaspoons marjoram

2 teaspoons thyme

1 tablespoon chives, minced (for garnish)

Grind the nuts in a coffee grinder until very fine.

In a large skillet, sauté the onions in oil on medium-high heat until translucent. Remove from heat and allow to cool slightly.

Transfer the nuts and onions to a blender with remaining ingredients and blend until smooth.

Transfer to a soup pot and simmer on medium heat for 20–30 minutes. Serve warm, garnished with minced chives.

Serves 4.

Substitutions

I love almonds in this soup as well. Experiment with different types of nuts. If you desire a smoother soup, buy nuts without outer coatings like whole almonds have, such as cashews or slivered almonds. If you want a smooth almond soup, soak the almonds overnight, and remove the peel by rubbing them through your fingers in the morning. When using soaked almonds you may need less water; you will have to blend the soaked almonds instead of grinding them in the coffee grinder.

Nutritional Analysis per Serving			
Vitamin A	127.6 RE	Vitamin D	0.0 µg
Thiamin (B-1)	0.2 mg	Vitamin E	1.4 mg
Riboflavin (B-2)	0.1 mg	Calcium	88.7 mg
Niacin	1.7 mg	Iron	5.3 mg
Vitamin B-6	0.3 mg	Phosphorus	610.0 mg
Vitamin B-12	0.0 µg	Magnesium	189.6 mg
Folate (total)	50.2 µg	Zinc	4.0 mg
Vitamin C	6.0 mg	Potassium	773.4 mg

Healthy Tidbit
The herb marjoram is related to oregano, but is generally milder. Marjoram stems can be laid across charcoal in the barbecue grill to add a faint flavor to food. The flowers will attract bees and butterflies to your garden, and the seed heads will provide food to birds in the winter.

Quick Turkey Soup

PER SERVING: 121.0 CALORIES ~ 14.1 G PROTEIN ~ 13.0 G CARBOHYDRATE ~ 1.7 G FIBER ~ 1.2 G
TOTAL FAT ~ 0.2 G SATURATED FAT ~ 31.4 MG CHOLESTEROL ~ 774.9 MG SODIUM

I found this recipe on the Internet and only had to change a few ingredients to make it suitable for the anti-inflammation diet. Don't be afraid to experiment with it.

6½ cups nonfat organic chicken broth	2 tablespoons miso paste
1½ cups of water	2–3 cups cooked turkey, cubed
1 cup diced onion	1 cup cooked brown rice
1 cup diced carrots	3 tablespoons chopped fresh parsley
1 clove garlic, minced	

Heat ¼ cup broth in a large saucepan over medium heat.

Add onion and carrots. Sauté until carrots begin to soften, about 5 minutes. Add garlic and sauté for an additional minute.

Add remaining broth, water, miso paste, turkey, and rice. Simmer for 20 minutes. Sprinkle with parsley before serving.

Serves 6.

Substitutions
If you have extra vegetables in your refrigerator that need to be cooked, add them to this soup; that way, it becomes something different every time you make it. If you can tolerate tomatoes, they would be a great addition to this recipe.

Healthy Tidbit
Always try to eat in a relaxed atmosphere as opposed to in the car, on the run, or while talking on the phone. Stressful situations and stress in general stimulate the sympathetic nervous system and downregulate the parasympathetic nervous system. The parasympathetic system is responsible for digestion; if it is downregulated while you are eating, you will fail to digest your food properly. So remember to "rest and digest."

Nutritional Analysis per Serving			
Vitamin A	528.0 RE	Vitamin D	0.0 µg
Thiamin (B-1)	0.1 mg	Vitamin E	0.4 mg
Riboflavin (B-2)	0.1 mg	Calcium	29.5 mg
Niacin	4.3 mg	Iron	1.3 mg
Vitamin B-6	0.3 mg	Phosphorus	151.7 mg
Vitamin B-12	0.4 µg	Magnesium	34.9 mg
Folate (total)	11.4 µg	Zinc	1.1 mg
Vitamin C	5.8 mg	Potassium	278.8 mg

Raw Beet Soup

PER SERVING: 237.8 CALORIES ~ 4.5 G PROTEIN ~ 30.7 G CARBOHYDRATE ~ 8.4 G FIBER ~ 12.6 G
TOTAL FAT ~ 1.8 G SATURATED FAT ~ 0.0 MG CHOLESTEROL ~ 168.0 MG SODIUM

This recipe comes from the marvelous cook Erika Siegel, N.D., L.Ac.

3 medium organic beets (enough to obtain 1 cup juice)

1 pound organic carrots (enough to obtain 1 cup juice)

¼ cup chopped green onion

½ cup shredded green cabbage

1 teaspoon chopped dill

½ cup finely grated beets

1 large avocado, spooned into chunks

½ apple, thinly sliced

Put beets and carrots through juicer to yield one cup of each. (You can buy fresh juice at a health-food store or juice bar if you do not have a juicer.)

Place all ingredients except avocado, grated beets, and apple into the blender, and blend until smooth.

Chill until ready to serve. Serve cold garnished with avocados, beets, and apple.

Serves 2.

Healthy Tidbit

Dill aids digestion, reduces flatus, reduces hiccups, eases stomach pain, and can help with insomnia. I like to use dill to flavor fish, especially salmon.

Nutritional Analysis per Serving			
Vitamin A	1,812.8 RE	Vitamin D	0.0 µg
Thiamin (B-1)	0.1 mg	Vitamin E	1.2 mg
Riboflavin (B-2)	0.2 mg	Calcium	55.1 mg
Niacin	3.2 mg	Iron	1.8 mg
Vitamin B-6	0.3 mg	Phosphorus	70.3 mg
Vitamin B-12	0.0 µg	Magnesium	39.4 mg
Folate (total)	103.0 µg	Zinc	0.8 mg
Vitamin C	21.0 mg	Potassium	897.6 mg

Sweet Potato Soup

PER SERVING: 125.0 CALORIES ~ 2.8 G PROTEIN ~ 20.4 G CARBOHYDRATE ~ 3.1 G FIBER ~ 4.1 G TOTAL FAT ~ 0.5 G SATURATED FAT ~ 0.0 MG CHOLESTEROL ~ 336.6 MG SODIUM

When I took this soup to a party everyone raved about it. I bet your friends and family will rave about it, too. This is a great soup to make ahead of time and freeze in portion sizes for later use.

2 large or 3 small sweet potatoes or yams, cut into chunks (I like to use yams)

1 onion, diced

5 garlic cloves, minced

1 tablespoon organic cold-pressed olive oil

15-ounce can organic chicken broth

¼ cup milk substitute such as rice milk, or water

1 teaspoon wheat-free tamari

½ teaspoon grated fresh ginger

1 teaspoon thyme (or more if you desire)

Sea salt and pepper to taste

Steam the yams or sweet potatoes until they are soft. This can take up to 40 minutes. Sauté the garlic and onions in olive oil until the onions are soft and translucent; set aside until potatoes are finished.

Once the potatoes are cooked, allow them to cool slightly. Place all ingredients except the milk substitute in the blender, and blend.

Gradually add the milk substitute until soup has reached desired consistency. Serve immediately while still warm.

Serves 4.

Substitutions
Using water instead of milk substitute won't make much difference in taste in this recipe.

Healthy Tidbit
The yam was first cultivated in Africa more than ten thousand years ago. Yams can be used to treat arthritis, asthma, and spasms. Their natural plant estrogens may help various female complaints. They help to bind heavy metals in the body, thereby assisting in detoxification of tissues.

Nutritional Analysis per Serving			
Vitamin A	1,364.6 RE	Vitamin D	0.2 µg
Thiamin (B-1)	0.1 mg	Vitamin E	0.5 mg
Riboflavin (B-2)	0.1 mg	Calcium	70.7 mg
Niacin	0.7 mg	Iron	1.3 mg
Vitamin B-6	0.2 mg	Phosphorus	161.0 mg
Vitamin B-12	0.1 µg	Magnesium	22.9 mg
Folate (total)	8.5 µg	Zinc	0.3 mg
Vitamin C	5.7 mg	Potassium	411.8 mg

Tangy Coconut Soup

PER SERVING: 323.0 CALORIES ~ 40.7 G PROTEIN ~ 14.6 G CARBOHYDRATE ~ 0.8 G FIBER ~ 11.1 G
TOTAL FAT ~ 4.6 G SATURATED FAT ~ 98.7 MG CHOLESTEROL ~ 367.4 MG SODIUM

I love tom kha soup, but I know that the versions served at most Thai restaurants contain sugar. This recipe allows you to experience a similar taste without added sugar. Galanga root and lemongrass can be purchased at Asian markets and at some well-stocked gourmet groceries.

2 chicken breasts, cubed (about 1½ pounds meat)

½ red onion, sliced into very thin rings

2 teaspoons olive oil

Galanga root (optional)

3 stalks of lemongrass, cut into large chunks (for flavor, not to be eaten)

1 hot chili, minced and seeded, or 2 generous dashes of dried cayenne pepper

10 small mushrooms, sliced thin

1 cup filtered water

Juice of ½ medium lemon

2 teaspoons fish sauce

1 tablespoon plus 1 teaspoon honey

1 13.5-ounce can light coconut milk

In a medium saucepan, sauté the red onion and chicken until onions begin to soften.

Add all remaining ingredients except the coconut milk. Stir to combine. Simmer for 15 minutes.

Add coconut milk and simmer for another 15 minutes or until vegetables and chicken are finished cooking. Do not boil the coconut milk or it will separate.

Serves 4.

Substitutions

Adding kaffir lime leaves will increase the tangy flavor.

Healthy Tidbit

These days it seems that all foods contain sugar. Even many Thai restaurants— and other restaurants for

Nutritional Analysis per Serving			
Vitamin A	132.6 RE	Vitamin D	0.9 µg
Thiamin (B-1)	0.2 mg	Vitamin E	0.6 mg
Riboflavin (B-2)	0.4 mg	Calcium	18.1 mg
Niacin	21.2 mg	Iron	1.3 mg
Vitamin B-6	1.1 mg	Phosphorus	60.4 mg
Vitamin B-12	0.7 µg	Magnesium	58.8 mg
Folate (total)	16.5 µg	Zinc	1.5 mg
Vitamin C	37.6 mg	Potassium	745.0 mg

that matter—add sugar to many of their dishes. Sugar consumption in the United States has reached what I consider to be a pathological level. Soft drink consumption has risen 500 percent in the past fifty years. Half of all Americans drink soft drinks daily. Sugar has many ill effects on the body, one of which is to increase insulin levels, which ultimately leads to energy conservation and fat production, hence promoting weight gain.

10-Minute Avocado Soup

PER SERVING: 797.5 CALORIES ~ 26.7 G PROTEIN ~ 30.2 G CARBOHYDRATE ~ 17.6 G FIBER ~ 69.9 G TOTAL FAT ~ 6.2 G SATURATED FAT ~ 0.0 MG CHOLESTEROL ~ 329.1 MG SODIUM

This soup is easy to make, tastes great, and fills the stomach on a cool night.

2 medium ripe avocados

2 cups almond milk

½ teaspoon cumin

½ teaspoon ground ginger

½ teaspoon salt

1 clove garlic, minced

Mash avocados in a pan.

Add all remaining ingredients. Stir well until mixed fully. You may use an electric beater or blender for this step.

When the soup is well mixed, heat just enough to serve.

Serves 4.

Substitutions

Use any seasonings you desire to make this soup your own creation.

Healthy Tidbit

Nearly all of the calories from avocados come from fat, primarily monounsaturated fat. Because the fat they contain is a healthful kind, avocados are a great food for individuals wishing to gain weight. They help to nourish and build the blood and yin. Because of avocados' buttery texture, they can replace butter as a spread and can complement many different dishes.

Nutritional Analysis per Serving			
Vitamin A	53.3 RE	Vitamin D	0.0 µg
Thiamin (B-1)	0.3 mg	Vitamin E	1.1 mg
Riboflavin (B-2)	0.7 mg	Calcium	259.2 mg
Niacin	5.6 mg	Iron	4.7 mg
Vitamin B-6	0.4 mg	Phosphorus	589.7 mg
Vitamin B-12	0.0 µg	Magnesium	336.7 mg
Folate (total)	83.4 µg	Zinc	4.1 mg
Vitamin C	8.7 mg	Potassium	1,200.4 mg

Sweet Things

Baked Red Apples

PER SERVING: 104.3 CALORIES ~ 0.5 G PROTEIN ~ 27.5 G CARBOHYDRATE ~ 3.5 G FIBER ~ 0.3 G
TOTAL FAT ~ 0.0 G SATURATED FAT ~ 0.0 MG CHOLESTEROL ~ 2.5 MG SODIUM

This recipe, another one from Erika Siegel, N.D., L.Ac., is a delectable after-dinner treat. Slide the apples into the oven as you sit down to your meal, and dessert will be warm when you finish dining. They also taste great the next day cold.

1 apple, Fuji, Braeburn, Gala, or personal favorite

1 teaspoon maple syrup

Dash of cinnamon

10 raisins

Fresh lemon juice to taste

1 teaspoon filtered water

Preheat oven to 375° F.

Core apple. Peel skin off top third of apple and place in individual baking dish. Drizzle maple syrup, cinnamon, and raisins over apple.

Squeeze a little lemon juice on top and add 1 teaspoon of water.

Bake uncovered for about 1 hour, and serve warm. Serves 1.

Substitutions

You could easily use pears instead of apples and reduce the cooking time to 40 minutes.

Healthy Tidbit

This dessert works well for Thanksgiving or other holiday dinners, when we often eat more food than typical. And what do we do after dinner? We often sit sluggishly, watching TV. Television has played a major role in promoting inactive lifestyles. Results of a study conducted by Fung et al. and published in the *American Journal of Epidemiology* in 2000 indicated that the average number of hours of television watched in 1994 was significantly positively associated with obesity and LDL cholesterol levels (the bad cholesterol) and significantly inversely proportional to HDL cholesterol levels (the good cholesterol). After your holiday feast, encourage your family to join you on a brisk walk instead of plopping down in front of the football game.

Nutritional Analysis per Serving			
Vitamin A	7.0 RE	Vitamin D	0.0 µg
Thiamin (B-1)	0.0 mg	Vitamin E	0.0 mg
Riboflavin (B-2)	0.0 mg	Calcium	15.2 mg
Niacin	0.1 mg	Iron	0.3 mg
Vitamin B-6	0.1 mg	Phosphorus	20.6 mg
Vitamin B-12	0.0 µg	Magnesium	9.5 mg
Folate (total)	4.4 µg	Zinc	0.3 mg
Vitamin C	6.5 mg	Potassium	199.8 mg

Blueberry Upside-Down Cake

PER SERVING: 253.7 CALORIES ~ 3.8 G PROTEIN ~ 34.9 G CARBOHYDRATE ~ 3.0 G FIBER ~ 11.1 G
TOTAL FAT ~ 1.6 G SATURATED FAT ~ 35.3 MG CHOLESTEROL ~ 121.0 MG SODIUM

This is a fun party pleaser with a wonderful presentation. Who ever knew that a treat this decadent could enhance your health? But remember, even healthy sweets should be eaten sparingly.

4 tablespoons extra-virgin olive oil

¹/₃ cup plus 3 tablespoons organic brown rice syrup

1 ½ cup fresh organic blueberries

Sea salt to taste

1 cup spelt flour

1 teaspoon baking powder

¼ cup rice milk or soy milk

1 organic egg, beaten

Preheat oven to 350° F.

Warm 1 tablespoon oil with 2 tablespoons rice syrup over low heat until syrup is runny and easy to spread. Then spoon the mixture evenly over the bottom of a greased 1-quart soufflé dish.

Sprinkle the blueberries into the soufflé dish; add a sprinkle of sea salt and set aside.

Mix together remaining ingredients (including remaining oil and syrup) until you have a smooth batter. Carefully spoon the batter over the blueberries, making sure not to disturb them.

Bake about 40–45 minutes, or until center of cake springs back when touched gently. Remove from oven, run a sharp knife around the rim of the soufflé pan, and invert immediately onto a serving plate. Any blueberry mixture that might stick to the pan can be spooned onto the cake after it is plated. Serve warm.

Serves 6.

Substitutions

You can try different flours with this recipe. When using a gluten-free flour, remember to add a binder such as ½ banana, ground flaxseeds, or arrowroot powder.

Nutritional Analysis per Serving

Vitamin A	19.6 RE	Vitamin D	0.1 µg
Thiamin (B-1)	0.1 mg	Vitamin E	1.5 mg
Riboflavin (B-2)	0.1 mg	Calcium	57.0 mg
Niacin	1.2 mg	Iron	1.1 mg
Vitamin B-6	0.0 mg	Phosphorus	40.5 mg
Vitamin B-12	0.1 µg	Magnesium	4.7 mg
Folate (total)	7.3 µg	Zinc	0.2 mg
Vitamin C	4.8 mg	Potassium	147.3 mg

Healthy Tidbit

Blueberries are a rich source of vitamin C and important bioflavanoids called proanthocyanidins, both of which are powerful antioxidants, meaning they protect the body from damaging, carcinogenic free radicals. Research conducted at Tufts University in 1996 rated blueberries number one in antioxidant activity among forty antioxidant-containing fruits and vegetables. This same research showed blueberries to diminish the effects of aging and improve memory.

Carrot Raisin Cookies

PER SERVING: 76.4 CALORIES ~ 1.4 G PROTEIN ~ 11.8 G CARBOHYDRATE ~ 1.0 G FIBER ~ 2.9 G
TOTAL FAT ~ 2.1 G SATURATED FAT ~ 6.0 MG CHOLESTEROL ~ 27.6 MG SODIUM

I modified this recipe from *The Complete Food Allergy Cookbook,* by
Marilyn Gioannini, M.D. Children like these cookies and at the same
time get their daily dose of beta-carotene. Using a combination of flours
and sweeteners makes these little treats even richer.

1½ cup spelt flour

1 cup oat flour

3 teaspoons aluminum-free baking powder

2 teaspoons cinnamon

2 teaspoons ground ginger

$2/3$ cup raisins (omit if you are diabetic)

½ cup chopped nuts (optional)

6 tablespoons coconut oil, warmed to a liquid consistency

3 tablespoons milk substitute (rice milk, soy milk, etc.)

1½ cup grated carrots

¼ cup raw honey (you may add 1 more tablespoon for a sweeter cookie)

¼ cup brown rice syrup (you may add 1 more tablespoon for a
sweeter cookie)

1 organic egg

Dash of salt

Preheat oven to 350° F. Mix together all dry ingredients, raisins, and
nuts.

In a large bowl, mix all wet ingredients together, including carrots;
gradually add the dry ingredients, making sure the raisins and carrots
don't clump together. For easier mixing, you can gently heat the honey
and brown rice syrup before adding them.

Drop with a spoon onto a greased baking sheet; bake for about 8
minutes.

Makes about 35–40 cookies.

Substitutions

You could add many different goodies to this recipe. How about some coconut, mixed nuts (except

Nutritional Analysis per Serving			
Vitamin A	135.9 RE	Vitamin D	0.0 µg
Thiamin (B-1)	0.0 mg	Vitamin E	0.1 mg
Riboflavin (B-2)	0.0 mg	Calcium	14.4 mg
Niacin	0.3 mg	Iron	0.5 mg
Vitamin B-6	0.0 mg	Phosphorus	22.5 mg
Vitamin B-12	0.0 µg	Magnesium	6.8 mg
Folate (total)	2.7 µg	Zinc	0.1 mg
Vitamin C	0.6 mg	Potassium	77.6 mg

peanuts), seeds, or a small amount of cut fruit? If you want to use a different flour, you could substitute quinoa or amaranth flour in place of the spelt flour. Remember to add ⅛–¼ cup of arrowroot powder or other binder.

Healthy Tidbit

Ginger has a long history of medicinal use in China and Japan. It has been used for treating simple nausea, other stomach complaints, colds, and headaches. Ginger is a very warming herb and can be helpful to someone who has a chilly constitution. Its anti-inflammatory properties make it helpful for rheumatic complaints.

Chunky Applesauce

PER SERVING: 76.4 CALORIES ~ 0.4 G PROTEIN ~ 20.4 G CARBOHYDRATE ~ 3.7 G FIBER ~ 0.3 G
TOTAL FAT ~ 0.1 G SATURATED FAT ~ 0.0 MG CHOLESTEROL ~ 1.8 MG SODIUM

My grandmother used to make homemade applesauce for us, and it was
my favorite.

8 fresh apples, peeled and cut into chunks (I prefer fujis because of their
sweetness)

2 tablespoons cinnamon

½ teaspoon nutmeg or to taste

1 tablespoon pure maple syrup (optional)

Place peeled, cut apples in a large saucepan with a lid. Add just enough
filtered water to cover the bottom of the pan. Cover and simmer on
medium heat for 5 minutes. Make sure the water does not evaporate,
and if you need to add more, do so sparingly.

Add cinnamon and nutmeg. Continue cooking, stirring often, until
apples are mushy, yet still have chunks, and the applesauce is to your
desired consistency.

Taste while warm; add maple syrup if you desire more sweetness.
With good apples, you shouldn't have to add the maple syrup.

Serves 8.

Substitutions
You could add some pears or peaches for a different flavor. For holiday
dinners you could add a small amount of beets or beet juice to make a
nice pink applesauce.

Healthy Tidbit
Apples have acids that inhibit fermentation in the stomach; therefore
they are easier to digest than many other fruits. Apples can quench thirst,
and they can clean your teeth if eaten after a meal. Green apples stimulate liver function and may
help to soften gallstones.
The pectin from apples
helps to promote growth of
healthy intestinal bacteria,
thereby aiding in gastro-
intestinal defense and
supporting healthy colon
function.

Nutritional Analysis per Serving			
Vitamin A	7.3 RE	Vitamin D	0.0 µg
Thiamin (B-1)	0.0 mg	Vitamin E	0.0 mg
Riboflavin (B-2)	0.0 mg	Calcium	29.2 mg
Niacin	0.1 mg	Iron	0.8 mg
Vitamin B-6	0.1 mg	Phosphorus	16.3 mg
Vitamin B-12	0.0 µg	Magnesium	7.9 mg
Folate (total)	4.7 µg	Zinc	0.1 mg
Vitamin C	6.8 mg	Potassium	156.3 mg

Coconut Vanilla "Ice Cream"

PER SERVING: 201.4 CALORIES ~ 2.8 G PROTEIN ~ 17.6 G CARBOHYDRATE ~ 0.7 G FIBER ~ 14.2 G
TOTAL FAT ~ 12.2 G SATURATED FAT ~ 0.0 MG CHOLESTEROL ~ 35.1 MG SODIUM

This recipe requires an ice cream maker.

1 13.5-ounce can coconut milk

1¼ cup vanilla soy milk

¼ cup honey

1 tablespoon vanilla extract

Combine all ingredients in a medium-sized bowl; mix well until honey is dissolved.

Turn ice cream maker on and pour mixture in.

Let ice cream maker operate for 30 minutes. Serve immediately.

Serves 6.

Substitutions

For even more flavor, add fruit or toasted coconut.

Healthy Tidbit

Chronic ear infections are commonly related to dairy allergy. Resolving chronic ear infections is often as simple as eliminating dairy from the child's diet. It was discovered as early as 1976 by Leonard Draper, M.D., that allergies as well as infection and mechanical blockage are important in the etiology of otolaryngology disorders.

Nutritional Analysis per Serving			
Vitamin A	31.3 RE	Vitamin D	0.5 µg
Thiamin (B-1)	0.0 mg	Vitamin E	0.0 mg
Riboflavin (B-2)	0.1 mg	Calcium	75.1 mg
Niacin	0.4 mg	Iron	2.5 mg
Vitamin B-6	0.0 mg	Phosphorus	114.0 mg
Vitamin B-12	0.0 µg	Magnesium	42.4 mg
Folate (total)	8.9 µg	Zinc	0.4 mg
Vitamin C	0.7 mg	Potassium	204.9 mg

Frozen Bananas

PER SERVING: 200.7 CALORIES ~ 2.2 G PROTEIN ~ 38.6 G CARBOHYDRATE ~ 7.4 G FIBER ~ 7.1 G
TOTAL FAT ~ 6.1 G SATURATED FAT ~ 0.0 MG CHOLESTEROL ~ 7.6 MG SODIUM

These are the perfect summer treat. Make many at once and keep them in the freezer for you or your children whenever a sweet craving strikes. If you have something healthy on hand, you are much less likely to binge on food that is not good for you.

1 ripe banana, cut into thirds

1 tablespoon carob powder

¼ teaspoon water

½ teaspoon honey

¼ cup unsweetened coconut, ground medium

In a small saucepan over medium-low heat, combine carob powder and enough water to make a paste. Add honey, and heat to desired consistency. Make sure it is not too runny.

Coat each piece of banana in carob mixture and roll in coconut. Wrap individually and place in the freezer until completely frozen (at least 30 minutes).

Take them out of the freezer 20 minutes before serving.

Serves 1.

Substitutions
These are a delicious, healthful alternative to chocolate, ice cream, or popsicles. Experiment with rolling them in different kinds of ground nuts or seeds.

Healthy Tidbit
Carob is alkaline in nature, nourishes the lungs, and is a great source of calcium. It also contains potassium, vitamin A, and vitamin B-complex. It contains 8 percent protein and has less fat and fewer calories than chocolate. It is free of caffeine, unlike chocolate, and is naturally sweet.

Nutritional Analysis per Serving			
Vitamin A	9.5 RE	Vitamin D	0.0 µg
Thiamin (B-1)	0.1 mg	Vitamin E	0.0 mg
Riboflavin (B-2)	0.1 mg	Calcium	31.2 mg
Niacin	1.0 mg	Iron	1.0 mg
Vitamin B-6	0.5 mg	Phosphorus	53.8 mg
Vitamin B-12	0.0 µg	Magnesium	41.8 mg
Folate (total)	30.7 µg	Zinc	0.5 mg
Vitamin C	11.0 mg	Potassium	548.4 mg

Ginger Snaps

PER SERVING: 201.4 CALORIES ~ 1.7 G PROTEIN ~ 29.7 G CARBOHYDRATE ~ 1.7 G FIBER ~ 9.2 G
TOTAL FAT ~ 7.7 G SATURATED FAT ~ 0.0 MG CHOLESTEROL ~ 248.7 MG SODIUM

Ginger snaps have been a favorite of mine since I was a little girl. This is a recipe from my friend and colleague Matt Fisel, N.D.

1½ cup tapioca flour

1 cup rye flour

½ teaspoon guar gum

1 teaspoon baking powder

1 teaspoon baking soda

½ teaspoon salt

¼ cup maple syrup

¼ cup brown rice syrup

½ cup coconut oil, warmed to a liquid consistency

5 tablespoons grated fresh ginger

Preheat oven to 350° F.

In a large bowl, stir together the flours, guar gum, baking powder, baking soda, and salt. Add the maple syrup, brown rice syrup, oil, and ginger. Stir together gently until just mixed.

Scoop spoon-sized portions onto a lightly greased cookie sheet and bake for 12–15 minutes.

Makes about 12 cookies.

Substitutions

You can add raisins to this recipe.

Healthy Tidbit

Brown rice syrup is a very versatile sweetener. It is nearly as sweet as honey and about twice as sweet as sugar; therefore, when you use it in baking, you need to use only half the quantity that you would use of white sugar. After a while, you'll come to know and love the sweeteners that are allowed on the anti-inflammation diet, and you won't even remember missing white sugar.

Nutritional Analysis per Serving

Vitamin A	0.0 RE	Vitamin D	0.0 µg
Thiamin (B-1)	0.0 mg	Vitamin E	0.3 mg
Riboflavin (B-2)	0.0 mg	Calcium	37.7 mg
Niacin	0.5 mg	Iron	1.0 mg
Vitamin B-6	0.1 mg	Phosphorus	83.1 mg
Vitamin B-12	0.0 µg	Magnesium	28.8 mg
Folate (total)	6.7 µg	Zinc	0.9 mg
Vitamin C	0.2 mg	Potassium	107.4 mg

Ginger Spice Cookies

PER SERVING: 183.0 CALORIES ~ 3.3 G PROTEIN ~ 25.7 G CARBOHYDRATE ~ 2.7 G FIBER ~ 8.4 G
TOTAL FAT ~ 6.0 G SATURATED FAT ~ 13.2 MG CHOLESTEROL ~ 150.7 MG SODIUM

These yummy treats have a cake-like consistency and texture. The recipe comes from Cyndi Stuart of Sheridan, Oregon.

1 cup brown rice flour	1 teaspoon cinnamon
1 cup rye flour	½ cup coconut oil, warmed to a liquid consistency
¼ teaspoon salt	
1 teaspoon baking soda	¼ cup real maple syrup
1 teaspoon baking powder	¼ cup raw honey
¼ teaspoon ground cloves (more if you like a strong clove flavor)	1 organic egg
	2 cups old-fashioned oats
1 teaspoon ground ginger	

Preheat oven to 375° F.

Sift together the first 8 ingredients and set aside.

Mix the oil, syrup, honey, and egg with an electric mixer on the lowest speed until well blended. With the mixer set on low speed, gradually add the dry ingredients to the wet; mix well.

Using a spatula, fold in the oats one cup at a time until incorporated. Drop dough by tablespoons onto an oiled baking sheet.

Bake for 8–10 minutes.

Makes about 16 cookies.

Substitutions

You might try different flours if rice and rye are not available.

Healthy Tidbit

Rye's health benefits mimic its heartiness as a crop. Rye helps to build muscles, promote energy, and support hepatic (liver) function. Nutritionally, rye is similar to wheat, but it contains significantly less gluten. Rye contains B vitamins, vitamin E, protein, and iron. Because of its gluten content, rye should be carefully rotated in the diet.

Nutritional Analysis per Serving			
Vitamin A	11.0 RE	Vitamin D	0.0 µg
Thiamin (B-1)	0.1 mg	Vitamin E	0.3 mg
Riboflavin (B-2)	0.0 mg	Calcium	28.8 mg
Niacin	0.4 mg	Iron	1.4 mg
Vitamin B-6	0.1 mg	Phosphorus	109.7 mg
Vitamin B-12	0.0 µg	Magnesium	48.6 mg
Folate (total)	10.5 µg	Zinc	1.0 mg
Vitamin C	0.1 mg	Potassium	114.2 mg

Hearty Healthy Cookies

PER SERVING: 186.8 CALORIES ~ 3.1 G PROTEIN ~ 19.2 G CARBOHYDRATE ~ 0.9 G FIBER ~ 11.5 G
TOTAL FAT ~ 6.4 G SATURATED FAT ~ 18.2 MG CHOLESTEROL ~ 175.1 MG SODIUM

These cookies were my first experiment with anti-inflammatory baking.
They have a great flavor and a lot of fiber.

1 organic egg, beaten	1 teaspoon baking soda
¼ cup rice milk	1 teaspoon cinnamon
½ cup organic butter (1 stick), softened	1 teaspoon sea salt
½ cup coconut oil, warmed to a liquid consistency	3 cups rolled oats
	½ cup walnut pieces
½ cup pure honey	¼ cup sunflower seeds
1 teaspoon vanilla extract	½ cup minced, peeled apple
1½ cups oat flour	

Preheat oven to 375° F.

Mix together wet ingredients, including softened butter, in a large
bowl. In a separate, smaller bowl, mix together flour, baking soda, cinnamon, and sea salt. Slowly add dry ingredients to wet ingredients, stirring constantly, until you have a smooth batter. Add oats, nuts, seeds,
and apple, stirring gently until mixture is uniform. Drop with a spoon
onto a greased cookie sheet, and bake for 9–12 minutes.

Makes 25–30 cookies.

Substitutions

If you cannot tolerate any dairy, coconut oil can be used instead of butter with no change in flavor. Any nuts or seeds and many fruits can be
used, so don't be afraid to experiment. Add grated zucchini to moisten
and add flavor to these cookies.

Healthy Tidbit

According to a randomized study published in the December 2004 issue
of *Diabetes Care,* adding walnuts to a low-fat diet improves lipid profiles for patients with type-
II diabetes. Walnuts are
distinguished from other
nuts by their higher polyunsaturated fat content (and,
importantly, their alpha-
linolenic acid [ALA] con-
tent) combined with their
high antioxidant content.

Nutritional Analysis per Serving			
Vitamin A	26.8 RE	Vitamin D	0.1 µg
Thiamin (B-1)	0.1 mg	Vitamin E	0.0 mg
Riboflavin (B-2)	0.0 mg	Calcium	16.1 mg
Niacin	0.4 mg	Iron	0.9 mg
Vitamin B-6	0.0 mg	Phosphorus	84.3 mg
Vitamin B-12	0.0 µg	Magnesium	18.6 mg
Folate (total)	9.1 µg	Zinc	0.4 mg
Vitamin C	0.2 mg	Potassium	84.5 mg

Mochi with Yogurt

PER SERVING: 367.6 CALORIES ~ 5.9 G PROTEIN ~ 82.4 G CARBOHYDRATE ~ 3.3 G FIBER ~ 1.4 G
TOTAL FAT ~ 0.2 G SATURATED FAT ~ 0.0 MG CHOLESTEROL ~ 23.8 MG SODIUM

This is a simple-to-make, not-too-sweet dessert. Mochi, originally a Japanese food, is pressed brown rice.

1 12.5-ounce package mochi (can be found in the refrigerated section of a health-food store)

1 cup plain soy yogurt
1 cup blueberries
½ cup pure maple syrup

Preheat oven to 350° F.

Cut mochi patty into 12 pieces and arrange on lightly greased baking pan. Bake until they begin to puff up and fill with air, about 12–16 minutes. Remove from oven. Top with yogurt and blueberries, and drizzle with maple syrup. Serve immediately.

Serves 4.

Substitutions

You can use any fruit instead of blueberries. I sometimes stuff the bite-sized mochi pieces with raisins or figs before baking, and then top with yogurt and syrup.

Healthy Tidbit

Japanese women are only one-third as likely to get breast cancer as American women. Genetics really can't account for the difference because when Japanese women migrate to the United States, their risk for breast cancer increases. So what is the difference between these two populations? Along with many health experts, I believe it is diet and lifestyle. Many American foods are low in quality and include artificial additives and fillers; the typical American diet consists of large amounts of refined and processed foods. As processed foods and fast foods have become more available in Japan, breast cancer rates there have increased (Japanese women used to have only one-fifth the risk of American women for developing the disease). Researchers have found that diets lower in total fat and lifestyles that include moderate exercise are protective against breast cancer.

Nutritional Analysis per Serving			
Vitamin A	3.6 RE	Vitamin D	0.0 µg
Thiamin (B-1)	0.1 mg	Vitamin E	0.4 mg
Riboflavin (B-2)	0.0 mg	Calcium	107.7 mg
Niacin	0.8 mg	Iron	1.0 mg
Vitamin B-6	0.1 mg	Phosphorus	22.2 mg
Vitamin B-12	0.0 µg	Magnesium	17.9 mg
Folate (total)	4.1 µg	Zinc	2.5 mg
Vitamin C	4.7 mg	Potassium	133.0 mg

No-Bake Oatmeal Cookies

PER SERVING: 181.1 CALORIES ~ 5.0 G PROTEIN ~ 25.1 G CARBOHYDRATE ~ 2.8 G FIBER ~ 7.6 G
TOTAL FAT ~ 0.8 G SATURATED FAT ~ 0.0 MG CHOLESTEROL ~ 53.3 MG SODIUM

I love to munch on these cookies, but I do so sparingly. They are good
for special occasions. It is better to eat these than to binge on white
flour, white sugar, or processed baked goods.

½ cup honey

½ cup brown rice syrup

3 cups oats

3 teaspoons carob powder

2 teaspoons vanilla extract

¼ cup melted organic butter (optional)

1 cup organic almond butter

Mix all ingredients together, form into cookie shapes, arrange them on
wax paper, and place in refrigerator to cool. Once cookies have cooled,
you can store them in an airtight container in the refrigerator.

Makes about 24 cookies.

Substitutions
You can use 1 cup honey or 1 cup brown rice syrup if you only have one
or the other. You can add many different goodies to this recipe. How
about some coconut, mixed nuts (except peanuts), seeds, a small amount
of cut fruit, or anything else you desire. If you are worried about calories, omit the butter.

Healthy Tidbit
Spending time in the kitchen may be new to you or it may be a favorite
pastime, but whatever the case, try to enjoy the experience. Instead of
dreading having to cook and prepare meals, reflect on the nature of the
food you are eating and use this time as a stress reliever. If you learn to
relax in the kitchen, your
cooking will improve, you
will digest your food properly, and you will find relief
from stress (which should
be a daily practice). Stress
relief is important for overall health, so most of all,
have fun.

Nutritional Analysis per Serving			
Vitamin A	0.0 RE	Vitamin D	0.0 µg
Thiamin (B-1)	0.2 mg	Vitamin E	0.9 mg
Riboflavin (B-2)	0.1 mg	Calcium	40.9 mg
Niacin	0.5 mg	Iron	1.4 mg
Vitamin B-6	0.0 mg	Phosphorus	157.5 mg
Vitamin B-12	0.0 µg	Magnesium	66.7 mg
Folate (total)	18.0 µg	Zinc	1.1 mg
Vitamin C	0.1 mg	Potassium	173.7 mg

Quick Sherbet

PER SERVING: 46.1 CALORIES ~ 0.9 G PROTEIN ~ 11.2 G CARBOHYDRATE ~ 1.7 G FIBER ~ 0.3 G
TOTAL FAT ~ 0.0 G SATURATED FAT ~ 0.0 MG CHOLESTEROL ~ 7.5 MG SODIUM

My husband and I were craving dessert one night, and all we had were some blackberries that I'd recently picked and frozen. I thought I'd blend them into a sherbet, and it worked! The benefits of experimenting come through again. The recipe may seem similar to a smoothie, but it really does come out like sherbet.

2 cups frozen organic strawberries (you can use almost any fruit, but berries work best)

¼ cup rice milk

2 tablespoons honey (optional)

Mint sprig (optional)

Put the frozen fruit in the blender and add the rice milk. Use just enough rice milk to get your blender going. If necessary, use a little bit more or less.

Add sweetener if desired, and blend until the the mixture reaches a smooth, sherbetlike consistency.

Garnish with a mint sprig and serve immediately.

Serves 4.

Substitutions
This simple recipe can work with many different fruits. You can use brown rice syrup or maple syrup instead of honey. Get creative when serving. You can hollow out a lemon and spoon the sherbet into the rind to serve it.

Healthy Tidbit
Mint, or *mentha,* has many uses. It is cooling, relieves abdominal pressure after a meal, and can defend against pathogens. Mint's aromatic quality invigorates the system by increasing circulation of blood, lymph, and energy. Mint is a great herb with which to garnish summer dishes and desserts since it cools and calms the temperament.

Nutritional Analysis per Serving			
Vitamin A	4.4 RE	Vitamin D	0.0 µg
Thiamin (B-1)	0.0 mg	Vitamin E	0.3 mg
Riboflavin (B-2)	0.0 mg	Calcium	20.2 mg
Niacin	0.5 mg	Iron	0.9 mg
Vitamin B-6	0.0 mg	Phosphorus	20.6 mg
Vitamin B-12	0.0 µg	Magnesium	14.6 mg
Folate (total)	20.2 µg	Zinc	0.2 mg
Vitamin C	45.5 mg	Potassium	180.3 mg

Sandy's Almond Butter Cookies

PER SERVING: 235.3 CALORIES ~ 2.6 G PROTEIN ~ 25.9 G CARBOHYDRATE ~ 0.7 G FIBER ~ 14.4 G
TOTAL FAT ~ 5.6 G SATURATED FAT ~ 38.0 MG CHOLESTEROL ~ 255.7 MG SODIUM

I have obtained many ideas about wheat-free cooking from my mother, Sandy Stock of Dubuque, Iowa, who has learned to survive with a wheat allergy in a wheat-inundated world.

¾ cup tapioca flour	½ cup organic butter, softened
½ cup rice flour	½ cup almond butter
¾ teaspoon baking soda	½ cup honey
½ teaspoon baking powder	1 organic egg
¼ teaspoon salt	

Preheat oven to 375° F.

Mix all dry ingredients together.

In a large bowl, mix butter, almond butter, honey, and egg; gradually add the dry ingredients. For easier mixing, you can gently heat the honey and butter before adding them to the mixture.

Drop with a spoon onto a greased baking sheet; bake for 9–12 minutes. Makes about 12 cookies.

Substitutions

These cookies taste just like peanut butter cookies. The tapioca flour adds a lightness to the batter. If you wish, you can use ¼ cup organic butter plus ¼ cup warmed coconut oil in place of the ½ cup butter.

Healthy Tidbit

Almond butter is a healthy source of protein. The recommended daily allowance for protein is as follows: A healthy male adult should consume 60 grams, a healthy female adult should consume 46 grams, and a child should consume anywhere from 16 grams to 28 grams depending on his or her weight and age. One cup of almonds contains 27 grams of protein, a chicken breast contains 30–40 grams, a can of tuna contains 24 grams, 3 ounces of salmon contains 21 grams, and 1 cup of refried beans contains 21 grams.

Nutritional Analysis per Serving			
Vitamin A	55.3 RE	Vitamin D	0.2 µg
Thiamin (B-1)	0.0 mg	Vitamin E	0.9 mg
Riboflavin (B-2)	0.1 mg	Calcium	46.9 mg
Niacin	0.4 mg	Iron	0.6 mg
Vitamin B-6	0.0 mg	Phosphorus	72.9 mg
Vitamin B-12	0.1 µg	Magnesium	32.9 mg
Folate (total)	9.4 µg	Zinc	0.4 mg
Vitamin C	0.1 mg	Potassium	95.5 mg

Sun Candies

PER SERVING: 115.2 CALORIES ~ 4.3 G PROTEIN ~ 4.9 G CARBOHYDRATE ~ 2.0 G FIBER ~ 9.6 G
TOTAL FAT ~ 1.0 G SATURATED FAT ~ 0.0 MG CHOLESTEROL ~ 5.9 MG SODIUM

Another name for these might be "esssential fatty acid candies" because they're chock-full of the stuff.

2½ cups sunflower seeds, ground in small batches in the coffee grinder

1½ tablespoons almond butter

1½ tablespoons raw honey

½ teaspoon vanilla extract

Mix together 2 cups ground sunflower seeds plus all remaining ingredients. Form into balls.

Roll balls in remaining ½ cup ground sunflower seeds to coat. Serve immediately; store in refrigerator.

Makes about 20 candies.

Substitutions
I like to roll the candies in coconut and/or carob power or add these ingredients to the recipe. You may need to increase quantities of almond butter or honey to get the balls to roll after adding coconut or carob powder.

Healthy Tidbit
One cup of sunflower seeds offers 10 grams of protein and almost 5 grams of fiber. Sunflower seeds are a great source of essential fatty acids and zinc, which is important in prostate health as well as for overall immune system health. Sunflower seeds are significantly high in magnesium, selenium, and folic acid.

Nutritional Analysis per Serving			
Vitamin A	0.9 RE	Vitamin D	0.0 µg
Thiamin (B-1)	0.4 mg	Vitamin E	0.1 mg
Riboflavin (B-2)	0.1 mg	Calcium	24.2 mg
Niacin	0.8 mg	Iron	1.3 mg
Vitamin B-6	0.1 mg	Phosphorus	133.2 mg
Vitamin B-12	0.0 µg	Magnesium	67.3 mg
Folate (total)	41.7 µg	Zinc	1.0 mg
Vitamin C	0.3 mg	Potassium	134.0 mg

Tahini–Almond Butter Cookies

PER SERVING: 121.1 CALORIES ~ 2.7 G PROTEIN ~ 17.3 G CARBOHYDRATE ~ 1.0 G FIBER ~ 5.0 G
TOTAL FAT ~ 0.6 G SATURATED FAT ~ 0.0 MG CHOLESTEROL ~ 119.2 MG SODIUM

This recipe came from one of my most diligent patients, Cyndi Stuart,
who has experimented on her own and has come up with some wonderful recipes.

2½ cups oat flour (I make my own by tossing oatmeal into the food
processor)

½ teaspoon baking powder

½ teaspoon baking soda

¾ teaspoon sea salt

½ cup sesame butter (tahini)

½ cup almond butter (no salt or sugar added)

1 teaspoon vanilla

½ cup brown rice syrup

¼ cup raw honey

¼ cup real maple syrup

Preheat oven to 350° F.

In a small bowl mix together all of the dry ingredients and set aside.

With an electric mixer, blend the two butters together until smooth.
If they become so thick that the mixer has trouble moving through them,
add filtered water, 1 tablespoon at a time, but no more than 4 tablespoons total.

Add the remaining wet ingredients, and beat on low speed until
blended.

Add the dry ingredients all at once, and beat together until well
blended. You may need to switch to a wooden spoon to finish the
mixing.

Drop by tablespoonfuls onto an oiled baking sheet. Bake until the
cookies are lightly brown
but still slightly soft, 10–12
minutes. Cool on a wire
rack and serve. Makes
about 24 cookies.

Healthy Tidbit

One important aspect of
baking is to make sure your

Nutritional Analysis per Serving			
Vitamin A	0.1 RE	Vitamin D	0.0 µg
Thiamin (B-1)	0.1 mg	Vitamin E	0.0 mg
Riboflavin (B-2)	0.1 mg	Calcium	35.8 mg
Niacin	0.4 mg	Iron	0.9 mg
Vitamin B-6	0.0 mg	Phosphorus	89.3 mg
Vitamin B-12	0.0 µg	Magnesium	33.3 mg
Folate (total)	8.5 µg	Zinc	0.7 mg
Vitamin C	0.1 mg	Potassium	98.6 mg

ingredients are as pure as you can find. For example, aluminum is added to many baking powders; to avoid it, it is vitally important to check labels and to purchase all-natural products when you have the option. And just because a product says it is "all natural" doesn't always mean it is good for you. Make sure to check labels for unhealthy ingredients.

An alternative to purchasing commercial baking powder is to make your own. Blend 2 parts cream of tartar, 1 part baking soda, and 2 parts arrowroot powder, and store in an airtight container. You can use this mixture in any recipe that calls for baking powder.

Substitutions Chart

Eliminated Food	Substitution	Directions
Cow's milk	Soy milk, rice milk, sesame seed milk, almond milk (or other nut milk), oat milk	Substitute equal quantities
Commercial eggs	Organic eggs are fine for some individuals. Or you can experiment with some of the following binders:	
	Flaxseeds soaked overnight in water or boiled for 15 minutes	1–2 tablespoons seeds in ½–1 cup of water
	Tofu, for scrambles or baked goods	¼ cup in place of 1 egg
	Banana, to bind baked goods (adds a sweet taste)	½–1 banana in cookies or muffins
	Arrowroot powder (use as a binder for nongluten flours)	1 tablespoon for each cup of nongluten flour
	Guar gum (you need only a very small amount)	¼–½ teaspoon for muffins, breads, and other baked goods
	Xantham gum	1 teaspoon for each cup of nongluten flour
Sugar	Honey (twice as sweet as processed cane sugar)	½ amount recipe calls for
	Pure maple syrup	½–¾ amount recipe calls for
	Brown rice syrup	½–¾ amount recipe calls for
	Stevia	Small amount; label will have conversions

Eliminated Food	Substitution	Directions
Wheat flour	When substituting these flours, you may want to add a little more baking powder or baking soda to help the baked goods rise.	
	Amaranth (can have a strong taste)	Needs a binder (see above)
	Barley (contains a small amount of gluten)	May need a binder
	Garbanzo	Needs a binder
	Kamut (contains gluten; should not be eaten every day)	No binder is needed
	Oat (may contain a very small amount of gluten)	May need a binder
	Quinoa (can taste bitter; should be mixed with other flours)	Needs a binder
	Rice (can be grainy; mix with other flours)	Needs a binder
	Rye (contains gluten; should not be eaten every day)	No binder is needed
	Soy (can have a beany flavor)	Needs a binder
	Spelt (contains gluten; should not be eaten every day)	No binder is needed
	Teff	Needs a binder
Potatoes	Yucca root, taro root, Jerusalem artichokes (sunchokes)	Cook similar to potatoes
Chocolate	Carob powder is nutritionally superior to chocolate	Substitute 3 tablespoons for 1 ounce chocolate
Butter	Blend of organic butter and olive oil (use as a spread) Blend of organic butter and coconut oil (use for baking) Nonhydrogenated vegan margarine spread	Substitute equal quantities
Peanuts, peanut butter	Almonds, almond butter	Substitute equal quantities

References

Airola, P. 1982. *Every woman's book*. Phoenix, AZ: Health Plus Publishers.

American Heart Association. 2003. Eating breakfast may reduce risk of obesity, diabetes, heart disease. *Journal Report,* March 6, http://www.americanheart.org/presenter.jhtml?identifier=3009715.

———. 2005. Dietary recommendations for children and adolescents: A guide for practitioners: Consensus statement from the American Heart Association. *Circulation* 112(13): 2061–2075.

Anderson, R. A. 2004. Autoimmunity and psychological states. *Townsend Letter for Doctors and Patients* 250:46–59.

Braly, J., and R. Hoggan. 2002. *Dangerous grains*. New York: Penguin Putnam Inc.

Bremness, L. 1994. *Herbs: The visual guide to more than 700 herb species from around the world*. New York: DK Publishing.

Centers for Disease Control and Prevention. 2004. The burden of chronic diseases and their risk factors: National and state perspectives. http://www.cdc.gov/nccdphp/burdenbook2004/.

Ciubotaru, I., Y. S. Lee, and R. C. Wander. 2003. Dietary fish oil decreases C-reactive protein, interleukin-6, and triacyglycerol to HDL-cholesterol ratio in postmenopausal women on HRT. *The Journal of Nutritional Biochemistry* 14 (September): 513–21.

Cornell University. 2003. Too many sweetened drinks, from soda to lemonade, put children at risk for obesity, poor nutrition, study at Cornell finds. *Cornell News,* June 26, http://www.news.cornell.edu/releases/June03/sweetdrink.kids.html.

Dasa, Kurma. 1990. *Great vegetarian dishes: Over 240 recipes from around the world*. Los Angeles, CA: The Bhaktivedanta Book Trust.

DeNoon, Daniel. 2003. Sesame oil benefits blood pressure. *WebMD Medical News,* April 28, http://www.webmd.com/content/article/64/72269.htm.

Draper, W. L. 1976. Secretory otitis media. *Clinical Ecology* 176–178.

Food and Drug Administration. 2004. FDA issues public health advisory on Vioxx as its manufacturer voluntarily withdraws the product. *FDA News,* September 30, http://www.fda.gov/bbs/topics/news/2004/NEW01122.html.

Fung, Teresa T., et al. 2000. Leisure-time physical activity, television watching, and plasma biomarkers of obesity and cardiovascular disease risk. *American Journal of Epidemiology* 152(12): 1171–1178.

Gioannini, M. 1996. *The complete food allergy cookbook: The foods you've always loved without the ingredients you can't have!* Rocklin, CA: Prima Publishing.

Gorman, C., and A. Park. 2004. The fires within. *Time,* February 23, 38–46.

Gueniot, Gerard. 2003. Individualized medicine. Lecture delivered at Portland Art Museum, Portland, OR.

Hippisley-Cox, Julie, and Carol Coupland. 2005. Risk of myocardial infarction in patients taking cyclo-oxygenase-2 inhibitors or conventional non-steroidal anti-inflammatory drugs: population based nested case-control analysis. *British Medical Journal* 330 (June): 1366.

Hippisley-Cox, Julie, et al. 2005. Risk of adverse gastrointestinal outcomes in patients taking cyclo-oxygenase-2 inhibitors or conventional non-steroidal anti-inflammatory drugs: population based nested case-control analysis. *British Medical Journal* 331: 1310–1316.

Jenkins, David, J. A. 2003. Current dietary recommendations focusing on diets low in saturated fat have been expanded to include foods high in viscous fibers and plant sterols. *Journal of American Medical Association* 290: 502–10, 531–33.

Khan, Alam, et al. 2003. Cinnamon improves glucose and lipids of people with type 2 diabetes. *Diabetes Care* 26: 3215–18.

Kinderlehrer, Jane. 1971. *Confessions of a sneaky organic cook.* Emmaus, PA: Rodale Press.

Knowler, William, et al. 2002. Reduction in the incidence of type 2 diabetes with lifestyle intervention or metformin. *New England Journal of Medicine* 346 (6): 393–403.

Lin, Robert Y., et al. 2001. Interleukin 6 and C-reactive protein levels in patients with acute allergic reactions: an emergency department-based study. *Annals of Allergy, Asthma, and Immunology* 87(5): 412–416.

Lindlahr, Henry. 1975. *Philosophy of natural therapeutics.* Essex, England: The C.W. Daniel Company Limited.

Lindlahr, Henry. 1914. *Nature cure: Philosophy and practice based on the unity of disease and cure.* Chicago, IL: The Nature Cure Publishing Company.

Makino, Ayako, et al. 2003. Increased renal medullary H_2O_2 leads to hypertension. *Hypertension Journal* 42:25.

Marz, Russel. 1999. *Medical Nutrition from Marz,* 2nd ed. Portland, OR: Omni-Press.

Michels, Karin, et al. 2006. Preschool diet and adult risk of breast cancer. *International Journal of Cancer* 118(3): 749–754.

Moore, Helen, et al. 2000. Nutrition and the health care agenda: a primary care perspective. *Family Practice* 17(2): 197–202.

Mozaffarian, Dariush, et al. 2004. Dietary intake of trans fatty acids and systemic inflammation in women. *The American Journal of Clinical Nutrition* 79(4): 606–612.

Mozaffarian, Dariush, et al. 2004. Trans fatty acids and systemic inflammation in heart failure. *The American Journal of Clinical Nutrition* 80(6): 1521–1525.

National Cancer Institute. 2001. Questions and answers: Annual report to the nation on the status of cancer, 1973–1998; feature focuses on cancers with recent increasing trends. *National Cancer Institute Fact Sheets,* June 5, http://www.cancer.gov/cancertopics/factsheet/1998-annual-report-increasing-trends.

National Institutes of Health Office of the Director. 2004. NIH halts use of COX-2 inhibitor in large cancer prevention trial. *NIH News,* December 17, http://www.nih.gov/news/pr/dec2004/od-17.htm.

Ngai P. H., and T. B. Ng. 2003. Lentin, a novel and potent antifungal protein from shitake mushroom with inhibitory effects on activity of human immunodeficiency virus-1 reverse transcriptase and proliferation of leukemia cells. *Life Science* 73(26): 3363–3374.

Osiecki, Henry. 2004. The role of chronic inflammation in cardiovascular disease and its regulation by nutrients. *Alternative Medicine Review* 9(1): 35–53.

Pissorno, Joseph, and Michael Murray. 1998. *Encyclopedia of natural medicine.* Rocklin, CA: Prima Publishing.

Pradhan, Aruna D., et al. 2001. C-reactive protein, interleukin-6, and risk of developing type 2 diabetes mellitus. *Journal of American Medical Association* 286(3): 327–334.

Riedl, Marc, and Adrian Casillas. 2003. Adverse drug reactions: types and treatment options. *American Family Physician* (November 1): 1781–1791.

Rodriguez-Cabezas, M.E., et al. 2003. Intestinal anti-inflammatory activity of dietary fiber (plantago ovata seeds) in HLA-B27 transgenic rats. *Clinical Nutrition* 22 (October): 463–71.

Rubin, Jordan. 2004. *The maker's diet.* Lake Mary, FL: Siloam/Strang Communications.

Sabaté, Joan, et al. 2003. Serum lipid response to the graduated enrichment of a Step I diet with almonds: a randomized feeding trial. *American Journal of Clinical Nutrition* 77 (June): 1379–84.

Schlosser, Eric. 2002. *Fast food nation: What the all-American meal is doing to the world.* London: Penguin Books.

Schmidt, Michael. 1996. *Healing childhood ear infections.* Berkeley, CA: North Atlantic Books.

Schulze, Matthias B., et al. 2005. Dietary pattern, inflammation, and incidence of type 2 diabetes in women. *American Journal of Clinical Nutrition* 82(3): 675–684.

Schwartz, Robert P. 2003. Soft drinks taste good, but the calories count. *Journal of Pediatrics* 142 (June): 599–600.

Shikany, James, and George White, Jr. 2000. Dietary guidelines for chronic disease prevention. *Southern Medical Journal* 93 (2000): 1157–61.

Soil Association (U.K.). 2006. Organic foods in relation to nutrition and health: key facts. Soil Association Library, revised June 22, http://www.soilassociation.org/web/sa/saweb.nsf/89D058CC4DBEB16D80256A73005A2866/4156CFCC00A84E8C80256E6800584151?OpenDocument.

Thom, Dickson. 2003. *Biotherapeutic drainage using the UNDA numbers.* Beaverton, OR: JELD Publications.

Thom, Dickson. 2002. Cellular and intracellular drainage with UNDA numbers. Lecture delivered at Fifth Avenue Suites, Portland, OR.

Thom, Dickson. Cellular and intracellular drainage with UNDA numbers: Advanced level. Lecture delivered at Fifth Avenue Suites, Portland, OR.

Tilgner, Sharol. 1999. *Herbal medicine: From the heart of the earth.* Creswell, OR: Wise Acres Press.

Tufts University. 2000. Tufts' blueberries research continues to generate headlines. *Tufts e-news,* March 20, http://www.tufts.edu/communications/stories/032000BlueberriesMakeMoreHeadlines.htm.

U.S. Department of Agriculture. 2004. Equivalence ensuring the flow of safe meat, poultry and egg products across country borders. http://www.fsis.usda.gov/PDF/Slides_051204_Swacina.pdf.

Wilkinson L., A. Scholey, and K. Wesnes. 2002. Chewing gum selectively improves aspects of memory in healthy volunteers. *Appetite* 38:235–236.

Wood, Rebecca. 1988. *The new whole foods encyclopedia.* New York: Penguin Books.

Wootan, Margo. 1996. Trans fat spells double trouble for arteries: What the food labels don't tell you. *Center for Science in the Public Interest* (August 7), http://www.cspinet.org/new/transpr.html.

Yance, D. R., and A. Valentine. 1999. *Herbal medicine, healing, and cancer: A comprehensive program for prevention and treatment.* Chicago, IL: Keats Publishing.

Yamadal, Yuji, et al. 2005. Effects of bread containing resistant starch on postprandial blood glucose levels in humans. *Bioscience, Biotechnology, and Biochemistry* 69(3): 559–566.

Online Resources

Author's website, including contact info: www.afamilyhealingcenter.com

www.naturopathic.org — Website for the American Association of Naturopathic Physicians; contains a database of naturopathic physicians by state

www.cand.ca — Website for the Canadian Association of Naturopathic Doctors; contains a database of naturopathic physicians by province

www.oanp.org — The Oregon Association of Naturopathic Physicians

www.healthrecipes.com — A great source for simple recipes

www.pubmed.com — Search here for articles from medical journals

www.medscape.com — Another source for articles from medical journals and other reliable resources

www.nih.gov — Website for the National Institutes of Health; contains links to many pages discussing chronic illnesses, healthy lifestyles, etc.

www.cdc.gov — Centers for Disease Control and Prevention

www.soilassociation.org — Information about organic foods from the U.K.

www.ewg.org — Environmental Working Group site that offers information about environmental toxins and their health hazards

www.pfizer.com — Contains current research on their pharmaceuticals and ongoing drug trials

www.ncnm.edu — National College of Naturopathic Medicine, Portland, OR

www.bastyr.edu — Bastyr University (an accredited naturopathic college), Kenmore, WA

www.scnm.edu — Southwest College of Naturopathic Medicine, Tempe, AZ

www.bridgeport.edu/naturopathy — University of Bridgeport College of Naturopathic Medicine, Bridgeport, CT

www.ccnm.edu — Canadian College of Naturopathic Medicine, Toronto, ON, Canada

Index

Boldface page numbers refer to recipes located in the text.

TABLE OF CONTENTS

INTRODUCTION

The Joy of Slow Cooking

The **CROCK-POT®** slow cooker is one of the most popular appliances in today's kitchen—and for good reason. What other appliance allows you to start your preparations for dinner in the morning, then gives you the freedom to enjoy your day far from your kitchen and return home to a hot savory dinner? You can easily take a slow-cooked dinner to a potluck supper and keep it warm during serving. When you're entertaining, you can rely on your slow cooker to free up a burner or leave valuable oven space for another item on your menu—plus cleanup is quick and easy. No wonder slow cookers are loved by cooks across America.

The information that follows will help you get the most from your **CROCK-POT®** slow cooker. You'll learn what they do best and why. Discover important techniques that can produce more flavorful dishes or help you create low-fat meals. Learn the tricks to cooking roasts, rice, pasta, and even baked goods in your slow cooker.

INTRODUCTION

Better yet, this book is packed with more than 200 taste-tempting recipes your family is sure to love. From easy appetizers and hearty main dishes to hot soups, spicy chilies, and satisfying desserts, this book has a fabulous collection of winning recipes and valuable information.

Don't wait any longer to get started on a quick course in slow cooking. Soon you'll be putting all your new knowledge to work to prepare family-pleasing meals every day of the week.

Picking the right one

CROCK-POT® slow cookers are available in a range of sizes to fill a number of different needs.

Smaller units, those capable of holding anywhere from 1 to 3½ quarts, are the perfect size for singles, a couple, or empty nesters, or for serving dips or spreads.

While medium-size slow cookers (those holding between 3½ and 5 quarts) will easily cook enough food at a time to feed a small family, these sizes are also convenient for holiday side dishes or larger quantities of appetizers.

Large slow cookers are great for large family dinners, holiday entertaining, and potluck suppers. A 6- or 7-quart model is ideal if you like to make meals in advance. They can easily make enough for dinner tonight with plenty of leftovers for later in the week.

Keep the lid on

A slow cooker can take as long as 30 minutes to regain heat lost when the cover is removed. Only remove the cover when instructed to do so in the recipe. Generally, slow cookers need very little stirring. With heating coils wrapped around the outside of the appliance and low heat, there's no danger of scorched food.

If you can't resist the urge to peek in the slow cooker, simply tap the cover gently or spin it lightly to remove condensation. You should be able to see what's going on in the slow cooker.

Filling the slow cooker

For best results, fill the slow cooker insert at least one-half full, but not more than three-quarters full. Many recipes recommend placing firm root vegetables on the bottom of the insert and the meat on top of the vegetables.

Make-ahead preparation

Mornings can be hectic times. If time is at a premium in the morning in your kitchen, you may find it easier to prep ingredients the night before. For safety's sake, cover and refrigerate all items until ready to use. Also, keep vegetables in a separate bowl from meat and poultry, and do not brown meat or poultry the night before to avoid other food safety issues. Just before cooking, add the prepared ingredients to the slow cooker; you may need to add an extra 30 minutes to the cooking time when using ingredients straight from the fridge as they will be very cold.

MAIN DISHES

Slow Cooking Main Dishes

Their ability to cook hearty, satisfying meals while largely unattended makes **CROCK-POT®** slow cookers tailor-made for today's busy families. Feeding your family a well-balanced meal is no more difficult than picking up a salad and a loaf of bread while your main dish, chock-full of lean meats and vegetables, is cooking itself on your kitchen counter.

Slow cooking is an effective way to tenderize meat, so tougher, less

MAIN DISHES

expensive cuts of meat (which have more flavor than lean cuts) are an excellent choice for slow cooking. Many of the recipes in the Main Dishes chapters include cuts like brisket, chuck roast, rump roast, stew meat, pork spareribs, and pork shoulder. But the selection isn't limited to just these cuts; you'll find some of the convenient choices you love, such as flank steak, ground beef, sausage, and pork chops.

It is best to trim meat and poultry of excess fat before cooking; the fat will liquefy and float to the top, and you'll need to skim it off after cooking. You may wish to brown meat in a skillet before adding it to the slow cooker *(see Browning below)*.

Browning

While not necessary, browning meat does have benefits. You've probably noticed that searing meat on a grill or in a skillet produces wonderful aromas and distinctive flavors that make steaks, burgers, and chops extra special. The flavor produced by browning will add complexity to slow-cooked beef, pork, and lamb meals. Ground beef and poultry should always be browned and drained of fat before it's placed in the slow cooker. Browning also gives meat a more pleasant color.

Buying fresh meat

In order to ensure that you are buying the freshest meat possible, look for packages that are securely wrapped with no signs of leakage, excess liquid or tears. The meat also should be cold to the touch. Choose fresh meat that has good color; avoid meat that is pale or gray-colored. Any fat should be firm and creamy white,

not yellow. The meat should have no odd odors. The surface should be moist but not slimy. Always check the "sell-by" date and only purchase on or before that date. Meat should only be purchased from a refrigerated case and should be securely wrapped and transported home quickly for immediate refrigeration. In addition, look for meat that is uniformly cut so it will cook evenly.

Beef

When choosing beef, look for: marbling, or flecks and thin streaks of fat that run throughout the piece of beef; a bright, cherry-red color (avoid meat with grayish tone or yellow fat); beef that is firm to the touch; and the cut. Loin and rib cuts tend to be more tender, while chuck, round, and flank tend to be less tender.

Pork

When choosing pork, look for moist meat that is pink in color (avoid meat with dry or discolored surfaces or a reddish or gray color); fat that is milky white; and the cut. Loin and leg cuts tend to be leaner. Lean cuts include tenderloin, loin chop, and sirloin roast.

(Check labels for cured or smoked pork cuts such as hams or sausage to see if the meat is "fully-cooked" or if it needs to be "cooked-before-eating.")

Preparing poultry

Chicken skin tends to shrivel and curl in the slow cooker, so most recipes call

It's easy to purchase skin-on chicken for greater savings and remove the skin yourself. Just grasp the skin using a paper towel and pull it away from the meat. The towel keeps the skin from slipping from your grip.

for skinless chicken. If you prefer to use skin-on pieces, brown them in a skillet before adding them to the slow cooker. Remove excess fat from poultry before cooking it.

Dairy products

Extended slow cooking (6 hours or more) can make dairy products curdle or separate. Add milk, cream, sour cream and cheese during the last 15 to 30 minutes of cooking.

Certain dairy products can be used successfully because they have undergone high heat processing. Examples of these are processed cheese and evaporated milk, which can be safely added early in the cooking process. Condensed soups—even cream-style varieties—can also withstand long cooking.

Boosting flavor

When most dried herbs and some spices are cooked for a long time they tend to lose flavor. As more steam condenses in the slow cooker and the liquid in the dish increases, flavors become diluted. (Conventional

MAIN DISHES

cooking, on the other hand, results in evaporation of liquid and seasonings tend to become stronger the longer they are cooked.) To correct this problem, always taste the dish about 30 minutes before the end of the cooking time and add additional herbs and spices as needed.

On the other hand, some spices increase in flavor with slow cooking. The best examples of this are black and red pepper, which can become very harsh and extra-spicy during long cooking. If you or a family member is sensitive to heat from pepper, use less than the recipe suggests or wait until the last 30 minutes to add it.

The flavors of fresh herbs will increase during long cooking, making fresh herbs a good choice for slow cooking.

Leftovers

Refrigerate leftovers quickly. Food can stand in a slow cooker that is turned off for up to 1 hour. To quickly chill leftovers, divide them into several small containers rather one large container; they will chill faster and give bacteria less chance to grow. Do not reheat leftovers in a slow cooker. Instead, heat them quickly on the top of the range or in a microwave oven.

BEEF

Braised Beef Brisket

2 tablespoons olive oil
1 beef brisket (3 to 4 pounds)
   Salt and black pepper, to taste
5 cloves garlic, minced
1 large yellow onion, diced
2 pounds Yukon Gold potatoes, peeled and cut into ¾-inch cubes
1 pound parsnips, peeled and cut into ¼-inch slices
1 pound carrots, peeled and cut into ¼-inch slices
1 cup red wine
1 cup beef broth
¼ cup tomato paste
1 teaspoon dried thyme
1 teaspoon dried rosemary
2 whole bay leaves

1. Heat oil in skillet over medium heat until hot. Season brisket with salt and pepper. Place garlic and onion in skillet. Brown brisket with garlic and onion, about 2 to 3 minutes per side. Transfer to **CROCK-POT®** slow cooker.

2. Add remaining ingredients and stir well to combine. Cover; cook on LOW 5½ to 7½ hours or on HIGH 3½ to 5½ hours or until meat is cooked through and tender.

3. Remove bay leaves before slicing and serving.

Makes 6 servings

Fiery Southwestern Enchiladas

STEAK FILLING

- 2 pounds tri-tip steak, cut into large chunks
- 1 cup water
- ½ cup tequila
- 5 cloves garlic, minced
- 1 serrano pepper, diced*
- 1 jalapeño pepper, diced*
  Kosher salt and freshly ground black pepper, to taste

ENCHILADA SAUCE

- 5 cans (7 ounces each) tomatillo sauce
- 1½ cups tomato sauce
- 1 pound Monterey Jack cheese, grated, divided
- 3 cans (15½ ounces each) black beans, rinsed and drained
- 1 can (8 ounces) corn, drained
- 16 flour tortillas
- 1 can (7 ounces) diced mild green chiles
- ½ cup sour cream (optional)
- 1 cup chopped fresh tomato
- ¼ cup chives, chopped

*Serrano and jalapeño peppers can sting and irritate the skin; wear rubber gloves when handling peppers and do not touch your eyes. Wash your hands after handling.

1. One day ahead, make the steak. Combine steak, water, tequila, garlic and peppers in **CROCK-POT®** slow cooker. Season with salt and pepper, to taste. Cover; cook on LOW 10 to 12 hours or until very tender. Shred steak. Refrigerate until ready to use.

2. Combine tomatillo and tomato sauces in saucepan over medium heat. Cook, stirring, until hot. Stir in ¼ cup cheese.

3. Heat beans and corn in another saucepan. Fill tortillas with sauce, beans, corn, cheese, steak, and diced green chiles, reserving ¼ cup each cheese, sauce and diced green chiles for topping. Roll tortilla and arrange in greased baking pan. Top with reserved sauce and sprinkle with reserved cheese and diced green chiles.

4. Cover pan with foil and bake 15 minutes in preheated 375°F oven. Top with sour cream, if desired, tomato and chives. Serve immediately.

Makes 8 servings

Classic Spaghetti

2 tablespoons olive oil
2 onions, chopped
2 green bell peppers, sliced
2 stalks celery, sliced
4 teaspoons minced garlic
3 pounds lean ground beef
2 carrots, diced
1 cup sliced mushrooms
1 can (28 ounces) tomato sauce
1 can (28 ounces) stewed tomatoes, undrained
3 cups water
2 tablespoons minced parsley
1 tablespoon dried oregano
1 tablespoon sugar
2 teaspoons salt
2 teaspoons black pepper
1 pound uncooked spaghetti

1. Heat oil in large skillet over medium-high heat until hot. Add onion, bell peppers, celery and garlic; cook and stir until tender. Transfer to **CROCK-POT®** slow cooker.

2. In same skillet, brown ground beef. Drain and discard fat. Add beef, carrots, mushrooms, tomato sauce, tomatoes with juice, water, parsley, oregano, sugar, salt and black pepper to **CROCK-POT®** slow cooker. Cover; cook on LOW 6 to 8 hours or on HIGH 3 to 5 hours or until done.

3. Cook spaghetti according to package directions; drain. Serve sauce over cooked spaghetti.

Makes 6 to 8 servings

Hearty Beef Short Ribs

2½ pounds beef short ribs, bone-in
1 to 2 tablespoons coarse salt
1 to 2 tablespoons black pepper
2 tablespoons olive oil, divided
2 carrots, cut into ¼-inch dice
2 celery stalks, cut into ¼-inch dice
1 large yellow onion, cut into ¼-inch dice
3 cloves garlic, minced
3 bay leaves
⅓ cup red wine
⅓ cup crushed tomatoes
⅓ cup balsamic vinegar

1. Season ribs with salt and black pepper. Drizzle with 1 tablespoon olive oil. Heat 1 tablespoon olive oil in large skillet. Cook ribs until just browned, about 2 to 3 minutes per side. Transfer ribs to **CROCK-POT®** slow cooker. Add carrots, celery, onion, garlic and bay leaves.

2. Combine wine, tomatoes and vinegar in small bowl. Season with salt and black pepper, if desired. Pour mixture into **CROCK-POT®** slow cooker. Cover; cook on LOW 8 to 9 hours or HIGH 5½ to 6 hours, turning once or twice, until meat is tender and falling off the bone.

3. Remove ribs from **CROCK-POT®** slow cooker. Process sauce in blender to desired consistency. To serve, pour sauce over ribs.

Makes 6 to 8 servings

Tip

For a change of pace from ordinary short rib recipes, ask your butcher for flanken-style beef short ribs. Flanken-style ribs are cut across the bones into wide, flat portions. They provide all the meaty flavor of the more common English-style short ribs with smaller, more manageable bones.

Fall Beef and Beer Casserole

- 2 **tablespoons oil**
- 1½ **pounds beef stew meat, cut into 1-inch cubes**
- 2 **tablespoons all-purpose flour**
- 1 **cup beef broth**
- 2 **cups brown ale or beer**
- 1 **cup water**
- 1 **onion, sliced**
- 2 **carrots, sliced**
- 1 **leek, sliced**
- 2 **stalks celery, sliced**
- 1 **cup mushrooms, sliced**
- 1 **turnip, cubed**
- 1 **teaspoon mixed herbs**

1. Heat oil in large skillet over medium-high heat until hot. Cook beef until browned on all sides. Transfer to **CROCK-POT®** slow cooker.

2. Sprinkle flour over contents of skillet. Cook and stir 2 minutes. Gradually stir in broth, ale and water (adding liquid ingredients too fast could create lumps in the sauce). Bring to a boil, and then pour over beef.

3. Add remaining ingredients to **CROCK-POT®** slow cooker. Cover; cook on LOW 8 to 10 hours or on HIGH 4 to 6 hours.

Makes 4 to 6 servings

Campfired-Up Sloppy Joes

1½ pounds lean ground beef
½ cup chopped sweet onion
1 medium red bell pepper, cored, seeded and chopped
1 large clove garlic, crushed
½ cup ketchup
½ cup barbecue sauce
2 tablespoons cider vinegar
1 tablespoon Worcestershire sauce
1 tablespoon packed brown sugar
1 teaspoon chili powder
1 can (8 ounces) baked beans
6 kaiser rolls, split and warmed
Shredded sharp Cheddar cheese (optional)

1. Brown ground beef, onion, bell pepper and garlic 6 to 8 minutes in large skillet over medium-high heat, stirring to break up meat. Drain and discard excess fat. Transfer beef mixture to **CROCK-POT®** slow cooker.

2. Combine ketchup, barbecue sauce, vinegar, Worcestershire sauce, brown sugar and chili powder in small bowl. Transfer to **CROCK-POT®** slow cooker.

3. Add baked beans. Stir well to combine. Cover; cook on HIGH 3 hours.

4. To serve, fill split rolls with ½ cup sloppy joe mixture. Sprinkle with Cheddar cheese, if desired, before topping sandwich with roll lid.

Makes 4 to 6 servings

Royal Round Steak

- 1 to 2 pounds round steak or stew meat cubes
- 1 to 2 tablespoons oil
- 1 envelope (1 ounce) dry onion soup mix
- 2 cans cream of mushroom soup
  Hot cooked egg noodles or cooked rice

1. Trim round steak and cut into cubes. (Partially freeze meat for easier cutting.)

2. Heat oil in large skillet over medium-high heat. Brown meat on all sides.

3. Combine dry soup mix and canned soup in mixing bowl. Pour into **CROCK-POT®** slow cooker. Add browned meat. Cover; cook on HIGH 6 to 7 hours.

4. To serve, spoon over prepared egg noodles or rice.

Makes 6 servings

Easy Beef Stroganoff

- 1½ to 2 pounds beef stew meat, cut into 1-inch cubes
- 4 medium potatoes, cut into 1-inch cubes
- 4 carrots, cut into 1½-inch pieces or 4 cups baby carrots
- 1 medium onion, cut into 8 wedges
- 2 cans (8 ounces each) tomato sauce
- 1 teaspoon salt
- ½ teaspoon black pepper
  Hot cooked egg noodles
  Chopped parsley, for garnish

Combine all ingredients except noodles in **CROCK-POT®** slow cooker. Cover; cook on LOW 8 to 10 hours or until vegetables are tender. Garnish as desired.

Makes 6 to 8 servings

Royal Round Steak

Suzie's Sloppy Joes

3	pounds 95% lean ground beef
1	cup chopped onion
3	cloves garlic, minced
1¼	cups ketchup
1	cup chopped red bell pepper
¼	cup plus 1 tablespoon Worcestershire sauce
¼	cup packed dark brown sugar
3	tablespoons prepared mustard
3	tablespoons vinegar
2	teaspoons chili powder
	Toasted hamburger buns

1. Cook and stir ground beef, onion and garlic in large nonstick skillet over medium-high heat until beef is browned and onion is tender. Drain and discard fat.

2. Combine ketchup, bell pepper, Worcestershire sauce, sugar, mustard, vinegar and chili powder in **CROCK-POT®** slow cooker. Stir in beef mixture. Cover; cook on LOW 6 to 8 hours. To serve, spoon mixture onto hamburger buns.

Makes 8 servings

Corned Beef and Cabbage

- **12 new red potatoes, quartered**
- **4 carrots, sliced**
- **1 corned beef brisket (about 4 pounds)**
- **2 onions, sliced**
- **3 whole bay leaves**
- **8 whole black peppercorns**
- **1 head cabbage, cut into wedges**

1. Place potatoes and carrots in bottom of **CROCK-POT®** slow cooker. Add brisket, onions, bay leaves and peppercorns. Add enough water to cover brisket. Cover; cook on LOW 4 to 5 hours or on HIGH 2 to 2½ hours.

2. Add cabbage. Continue cooking on LOW 4 to 5 hours longer or on HIGH 2 to 2½ hours longer. Slice brisket against the grain, and serve with vegetables.

Makes 6 to 8 servings

Philly Cheese Steaks

- 2 **pounds round steak, sliced**
- 2 **tablespoons butter or margarine, melted**
- 4 **onions, sliced**
- 2 **green bell peppers, sliced**
- 1 **tablespoon garlic-pepper blend**
  Salt, to taste
- ½ **cup water**
- 2 **teaspoons beef bouillon granules**
- 8 **crusty Italian or French rolls***
- 8 **slices Cheddar cheese, cut in half**

Toast rolls under broiler or on griddle, if desired.

1. Combine steak, butter, onions, green pepper, garlic-pepper blend and salt in **CROCK-POT®** slow cooker; stir to mix.

2. Whisk together water and bouillon in small bowl; pour into **CROCK-POT®** slow cooker. Cover; cook on LOW 6 to 8 hours.

3. Remove meat, onions and bell pepper from **CROCK-POT®** slow cooker and pile on rolls. Top with cheese and place under broiler until cheese is melted.

Makes 8 servings

Classic Beef and Noodles

- **1 tablespoon vegetable oil**
- **2 pounds beef for stew, cut into 1-inch pieces**
- **¼ pound fresh mushrooms, sliced into halves**
- **2 tablespoons chopped onion**
- **2 cloves garlic, minced**
- **1 teaspoon salt**
- **1 teaspoon dried oregano**
- **½ teaspoon black pepper**
- **¼ teaspoon dried marjoram**
- **1 bay leaf**
- **1½ cups beef broth**
- **⅓ cup dry sherry**
- **1 container (8 ounces) sour cream**
- **½ cup all-purpose flour**
- **¼ cup water**
- **4 cups hot cooked noodles**

1. Heat oil in large skillet over medium heat until hot. Brown beef on all sides. (Work in batches, if necessary.) Drain fat and discard.

2. Combine beef, mushrooms, onion, garlic, salt, oregano, pepper, marjoram and bay leaf in **CROCK-POT®** slow cooker. Pour in broth and sherry. Cover; cook on LOW 8 to 10 hours or on HIGH 4 to 5 hours. Remove bay leaf and discard.

3. Combine sour cream, flour and water in small bowl. Stir about 1 cup cooking liquid from **CROCK-POT®** slow cooker into sour cream mixture. Add mixture to **CROCK-POT®** slow cooker; mix well. Cook, uncovered, on HIGH 30 minutes or until thickened and bubbly. Serve over noodles.

Makes 8 servings

Best Beef Brisket Sandwich Ever

- **1 beef brisket (about 3 pounds)**
- **2 cups apple cider, divided**
- **1 head garlic, cloves separated, crushed and peeled**
- **2 tablespoons whole peppercorns**
- **1/3 cup chopped fresh thyme or 2 tablespoons dried thyme**
- **1 tablespoon mustard seeds**
- **1 tablespoon Cajun seasoning**
- **1 teaspoon ground allspice**
- **1 teaspoon ground cumin**
- **1 teaspoon celery seeds**
- **2 to 4 whole cloves**
- **1 bottle (12 ounces) dark beer**
- **10 to 12 sourdough sandwich rolls, sliced in half**

1. Place brisket, 1/2 cup cider, garlic, peppercorns, thyme, mustard seeds, Cajun seasoning, allspice, cumin, celery seeds and cloves in large resealable food storage bag. Seal bag; marinate in refrigerator overnight.

2. Place brisket and marinade in **CROCK-POT®** slow cooker. Add remaining 1 1/2 cups apple cider and beer. Cover; cook on LOW 10 hours or until brisket is tender.

3. Strain sauce; drizzle over meat. Slice brisket and place on sandwich rolls.

Makes 10 to 12 servings

Cocktail Meatballs

- 1 **pound 95% lean ground beef**
- 1 **pound bulk pork or Italian sausage**
- 1 **cup cracker crumbs**
- 1 **cup finely chopped onion**
- 1 **cup finely chopped green bell pepper**
- ½ **cup milk**
- 1 **egg, beaten**
- 2 **teaspoons salt**
- 1 **teaspoon dried Italian seasoning**
- ¼ **teaspoon black pepper**
- 1 **cup ketchup**
- ¾ **cup packed dark brown sugar**
- ½ **cup (1 stick) butter or margarine**
- ½ **cup vinegar**
- ¼ **cup lemon juice**
- ¼ **cup water**
- 1 **teaspoon prepared mustard**
- ¼ **teaspoon garlic salt**

1. Preheat oven to 350°F. Combine beef, pork, cracker crumbs, onion, bell pepper, milk, egg, salt, Italian seasoning and black pepper in bowl. Mix well; form into 1-inch meatballs. Place meatballs onto 2 nonstick baking sheets. Bake 25 minutes or until browned.

2. Meanwhile, place ketchup, sugar, butter, vinegar, lemon juice, water, mustard and garlic salt into **CROCK-POT®** slow cooker; mix well. Cover; cook on HIGH 15 to 20 minutes or until hot.

3. Transfer meatballs to **CROCK-POT®** slow cooker; carefully stir to coat with sauce. Reduce heat to LOW. Cover; cook 2 hours.

Makes about 24 meatballs

POULTRY

Spanish Paella with Chicken and Sausage

- 1 tablespoon olive oil
- 4 chicken thighs (about 2 pounds total)
- 1 medium onion, chopped
- 1 clove garlic, minced
- 1 pound hot smoked sausage, sliced into rounds
- 1 can (14½ ounces) stewed tomatoes, undrained
- 1 cup arborio rice
- 4 cups chicken broth
- 1 pinch saffron (optional)
- ½ cup frozen peas, thawed

1. Heat oil in large skillet over medium-high heat until hot. Add chicken pieces in batches and brown well on all sides. Transfer chicken to **CROCK-POT®** slow cooker as it browns.

2. Add onion to same skillet and cook until translucent. Stir in garlic, sausage, tomatoes with juice, rice and chicken broth. Stir in saffron, if desired. Pour over chicken. Cover and cook on LOW 6 to 8 hours or on HIGH 3 to 4 hours or until chicken is fully cooked and rice is tender.

3. Remove chicken pieces to serving platter and fluff rice with fork. Stir in peas. Spoon rice onto platter with chicken.

Makes 4 servings

Chicken Gumbo over Rice

 4 tablespoons olive oil, divided
 ½ pound Italian sausage, cut into ¼-inch slices
 ¼ cup all-purpose flour
 1 pound boneless, skinless chicken breasts,
    cut into ½-inch slices
 1 cup chopped onions
 1 cup chopped celery
 1 cup diced green bell peppers
 2 tablespoons minced jalapeño or serrano peppers*
 1 teaspoon paprika
1½ cups fresh or frozen okra, cut into ¼-inch slices
 1 cup chicken broth
 ½ cup white wine
 2 cups cooked brown or white rice

*Jalapeño and serrano peppers can sting and irritate the skin, so wear rubber gloves when handling peppers and do not touch your eyes.

1. Heat 2 tablespoons oil in skillet over medium heat until hot. Brown and crumble sausage until no pink remains, about 10 minutes. Transfer to paper towel-lined plate with slotted spoon to drain excess fat.

2. Heat remaining 2 tablespoons oil in skillet. Add flour and continuously stir with a whisk. Cook until flour becomes dark brown but not burnt. Add chicken, onions, celery, bell peppers, jalapeño peppers and paprika. Cook and stir 7 to 8 minutes, or until vegetables soften. Transfer to **CROCK-POT®** slow cooker.

3. Add drained sausage, okra, broth and wine. Cover; cook on LOW 7 to 8 hours or on HIGH 4 to 6 hours. Serve over cooked rice.

Makes 6 servings

Thai Coconut Chicken Meatballs

- 1 **pound ground chicken**
- 2 **green onions (white and green parts), chopped**
- 1 **clove garlic, minced**
- 2 **teaspoons toasted sesame oil**
- 1 **teaspoon fish sauce**
- 2 **teaspoons mirin**
- 1 **tablespoon canola oil**
- ½ **cup unsweetened canned coconut milk**
- ¼ **cup chicken broth**
- 1 **teaspoon Thai red curry paste**
- 2 **teaspoons packed brown sugar**
- 2 **teaspoons lime juice**
- 1 **tablespoon cornstarch**
- 2 **tablespoons cold water**

1. Combine chicken, green onions, garlic, sesame oil, fish sauce and mirin in large bowl. Mix well to combine and shape into meatballs about 1½ inches in diameter.

2. Heat canola oil in large skillet over medium-high heat. Add meatballs and cook, rolling to brown on all sides. Transfer to **CROCK-POT**® slow cooker. Add coconut milk, chicken broth, curry paste and sugar. Cover and cook on HIGH 3½ to 4 hours. Stir in lime juice.

3. Stir cornstarch into cold water, mixing until smooth. Stir in additional water as needed to reach consistency of heavy cream. Stir into sauce in **CROCK-POT**® slow cooker. Cook uncovered 10 to 15 minutes until sauce is slightly thickened and evenly coats meatballs.

Makes 4 to 5 servings

Tip

Meatballs that are of equal size will cook at the same rate and be done at the same time. To ensure your meatballs are the same size, pat seasoned ground meat into an even rectangle and then slice into even rows and columns. Roll each portion into smooth ball.

Tarragon Turkey and Pasta

1½ **to 2 pounds turkey tenderloins**
½ **cup thinly sliced celery**
¼ **cup thinly sliced green onions**
4 **tablespoons fresh tarragon, minced**
¼ **cup dry white wine**
1 **teaspoon salt**
1 **teaspoon freshly ground black pepper**
½ **cup plain yogurt**
1 **tablespoon fresh minced Italian parsley**
1 **tablespoon lemon juice**
1½ **tablespoons cornstarch**
2 **tablespoons water**
4 **cups pasta of your choice, cooked al denté**

1. Combine turkey, celery, green onions, 2 tablespoons fresh tarragon, wine, salt and pepper in **CROCK-POT®** slow cooker. Mix thoroughly. Cover; cook on LOW 6 to 8 hours or on HIGH 3½ to 4 hours or until turkey is no longer pink.

2. Remove turkey; cut into ½-inch-thick medallions. Turn **CROCK-POT®** slow cooker to HIGH. Stir yogurt, remaining 2 tablespoons fresh tarragon, parsley and lemon juice into cooking liquid.

3. Combine cornstarch and water in small bowl. Stir into cooking liquid and cook until thickened. Serve turkey medallions over pasta. Drizzle with tarragon sauce.

Makes 4 servings

Note
This easy dish is elegant enough to serve at a dinner party.

Tip
Recipe can be doubled for a 5-, 6- or 7-quart CROCK-POT® slow cooker.

Spicy Grits with Chicken

4	**cups chicken broth**
1	**cup grits***
1	**jalapeño pepper, cored, seeded and finely chopped****
½	**teaspoon salt, or to taste**
¼	**teaspoon paprika**
¼	**teaspoon black pepper, or to taste**
¾	**cup shredded sharp Cheddar cheese**
1½	**cups chopped cooked chicken breast (about 12 ounces)**
½	**cup half-and-half**
2	**tablespoons chopped chives, plus additional for garnish**

Use coarse, instant, yellow or stone-ground grits.

**Jalapeño peppers can sting and irritate the skin, so wear rubber gloves when handling peppers and do not touch your eyes.*

1. Combine broth, grits, jalapeño, salt, paprika and pepper in **CROCK-POT®** slow cooker. Stir well. Cover; cook on LOW 4 hours. (Consistency of cooked grits should be like cream of wheat.)

2. Add cheese and stir until melted. Stir in chicken, half-and-half and 2 tablespoons chives. Add salt and pepper, if desired. Cover; cook on LOW 15 minutes to blend flavors. Garnish with chives, if desired. Serve immediately.

Makes 6 servings

Chicken and Biscuits

4 boneless, skinless chicken breasts
1 can (10¾ ounces) condensed cream of chicken soup
1 package (10 ounces) frozen peas and carrots
1 package (7½ ounces) refrigerated biscuits

1. Cut chicken breasts into bite-size pieces. Place in **CROCK-POT®** slow cooker. Pour soup over chicken. Cover; cook on LOW 4 hours or until chicken is tender and no longer pink in center.

2. Stir in frozen vegetables. Cover and cook 30 minutes longer until vegetables are heated through.

3. Bake biscuits according to package directions. Spoon chicken and vegetable mixture over biscuits and serve.

Makes 4 servings

Lemon and Herb Turkey Breast

1   split turkey breast (about 3 pounds)
½   cup lemon juice
6   cloves garlic, minced
¼   teaspoon dried parsley
¼   teaspoon dried tarragon
¼   teaspoon dried rosemary
¼   teaspoon dried sage
¼   teaspoon salt
¼   teaspoon black pepper
½   cup dry white wine

1. Place turkey breast in **CROCK-POT®** slow cooker, adjusting turkey to fit as needed.

2. Combine remaining ingredients in small bowl. Pour over turkey breast. Cover; cook on LOW 8 to 10 hours or on HIGH 4 to 5 hours.

Makes 6 servings

Chicken and Biscuits

BBQ Turkey Legs

- **6 turkey drumsticks**
- **2 teaspoons salt**
- **2 teaspoons black pepper**
- **BBQ Sauce (recipe follows)**

Season drumsticks with salt and pepper. Place in **CROCK-POT®** slow cooker. Add BBQ Sauce, and turn drumsticks to coat evenly. Cover; cook on LOW 7 to 8 hours or on HIGH 3 to 4 hours. Enjoy hot or cold.

Makes 6 servings

BBQ Sauce

- **½ cup white vinegar**
- **½ cup ketchup**
- **½ cup molasses**
- **4 tablespoons Worcestershire sauce**
- **1 tablespoon onion powder**
- **1 tablespoon garlic powder**
- **1 teaspoon hickory liquid smoke**
- **⅛ teaspoon minced chipotle pepper**

Combine all ingredients and mix well. Proceed as directed above.

Makes about 2 cups sauce

BBQ Turkey Legs

Teriyaki Chicken Wings

- **3 to 4 pounds chicken wings**
- **¼ cup soy sauce**
- **¼ cup sherry**
- **¼ cup honey**
- **1 tablespoon hoisin sauce**
- **1 tablespoon orange juice**
- **2 cloves garlic, minced**
- **1 fresh red chili pepper, finely chopped* (optional)**

*Chili peppers can sting and irritate the skin, so wear rubber gloves when handling peppers and do not touch your eyes.

1. Place wings in **CROCK-POT®** slow cooker. Combine remaining ingredients in mixing bowl. Pour mixture over wings.

2. Cover; cook on LOW 3 to 3½ hours or on HIGH 1½ to 2 hours.

Makes 6 to 8 servings

Boneless Chicken Cacciatore

Olive oil
6 boneless, skinless chicken breasts, sliced in half horizontally
4 cups tomato-basil sauce or marinara sauce
1 cup coarsely chopped yellow onion
1 cup coarsely chopped green bell pepper
1 can (6 ounces) sliced mushrooms
¼ cup dry red wine (optional)
2 teaspoons minced garlic
2 teaspoons dried oregano, crushed
2 teaspoons dried thyme, crushed
2 teaspoons salt
2 teaspoons black pepper

1. Heat oil in skillet over medium heat until hot. Brown chicken on both sides, turning as it browns. Drain and transfer to **CROCK-POT®** slow cooker.

2. Add remaining ingredients, and stir well to combine. Cover; cook on LOW 5 to 7 hours or on HIGH 2 to 3 hours.

Makes 8 servings

Turkey Breast with Sweet Cranberry-Soy Sauce

1 **bone-in turkey breast, thawed, rinsed and patted dry (6 to 7 pounds)***

1 **can (16 ounces) whole berry cranberry sauce**

1 **packet (1 ounce) dry onion soup mix**
   Grated peel and juice of 1 medium orange

3 **tablespoons soy sauce**

2 **to 3 tablespoons cornstarch**

1 **to 1½ tablespoons sugar**

1 **to 1½ teaspoons cider vinegar**
   Salt, to taste

*Substitute 2 (3½-pound) bone-in turkey breast halves, if necessary.

1. Coat **CROCK-POT®** slow cooker with nonstick cooking spray. Place turkey in bottom, meat side up. Combine cranberry sauce, soup mix, orange peel and orange juice in small bowl. Pour over turkey. Cover; cook on HIGH 3½ hours.

2. Scrape cranberry mixture into cooking liquid. Transfer turkey to cutting board. Let stand 15 minutes before slicing.

3. Combine soy sauce and cornstarch in small bowl. Stir into cooking liquid with sugar, vinegar and salt, if desired. Cover; cook on HIGH 15 minutes longer, or until thickened slightly. Serve sauce over sliced turkey.

Makes 8 servings

Like Grandma's Chicken 'n' Dumplings

2 cups cooked chicken
1 can (10¾ ounces) condensed cream of mushroom soup, undiluted
1 can (10¾ ounces) condensed cream of chicken soup, undiluted
2 soup cans water
4 teaspoons all-purpose flour
2 teaspoons chicken bouillon granules
½ teaspoon black pepper
1 can refrigerated buttermilk biscuits (8 biscuits)

1. Mix all ingredients except biscuits in **CROCK-POT®** slow cooker.

2. Cut biscuits into quarters and gently stir into mixture. Cover; cook on LOW 4 to 6 hours.

Makes 4 to 6 servings

Chicken with Italian Sausage

- 10 **ounces bulk mild or hot Italian sausage**
- 6 **boneless, skinless chicken thighs**
- 1 **can (about 15 ounces) white beans, rinsed and drained**
- 1 **can (about 15 ounces) red beans, rinsed and drained**
- 1 **cup chicken broth**
- 1 **medium onion, chopped**
- 1 **teaspoon black pepper**
- ½ **teaspoon salt**
  Chopped fresh parsley

1. Brown sausage in large skillet over medium-high heat, stirring to break up meat. Drain fat and discard. Spoon sausage into **CROCK-POT®** slow cooker.

2. Trim fat from chicken and discard. Place chicken, beans, broth, onion, pepper and salt in **CROCK-POT®** slow cooker. Cover; cook on LOW 5 to 6 hours.

3. Adjust seasonings, if desired. Slice each chicken thigh on the diagonal. Serve with sausage and beans. Garnish with parsley.

Makes 6 servings

Greek-Style Chicken

- **6 boneless, skinless chicken thighs**
- **½ teaspoon salt**
- **½ teaspoon black pepper**
- **1 tablespoon olive oil**
- **½ cup chicken broth**
- **1 lemon, thinly sliced**
- **¼ cup pitted kalamata olives**
- **1 clove garlic, minced**
- **½ teaspoon dried oregano**
- **Hot cooked orzo or rice**

1. Remove and discard visible fat from chicken. Season chicken with salt and pepper. Heat oil in large skillet over medium-high heat until hot. Brown chicken on all sides. Transfer to **CROCK-POT®** slow cooker.

2. Add broth, lemon, olives, garlic and oregano. Cover; cook on LOW 5 to 6 hours or until chicken is tender. Serve with orzo.

Makes 4 to 6 servings

Tip
Freeze leftovers as individual portions; just reheat in a microwave for fast weeknight dinners!

PORK

Roast Ham with Tangy Mustard Glaze

1	**fully cooked boneless ham (about 3 pounds), visible fat removed**
¼	**cup packed dark brown sugar**
2	**tablespoons lemon juice, divided**
1	**tablespoon Dijon mustard**
½	**teaspoon ground allspice**
¼	**cup granulated sugar**
2	**tablespoons cornstarch**

1. Place ham in **CROCK-POT®** slow cooker. Combine brown sugar, 2 teaspoons lemon juice, mustard and allspice. Spoon evenly over ham. Cover; cook on LOW 6 to 7 hours, or until ham is warm throughout and sauce is well absorbed. Transfer ham to warm serving platter.

2. Pour cooking liquid from **CROCK-POT®** slow cooker into small heavy saucepan. Add remaining lemon juice, granulated sugar and cornstarch. Cook over medium-high heat until mixture boils. Reduce to medium heat. Cook and stir until sauce is thickened and glossy.

3. Carve ham into slices and spoon sauce over individual servings.

Makes 12 to 15 servings

Pork Roast with Fruit Medley

1 **cup water**
½ **cup kosher or coarse salt**
2 **tablespoons sugar**
1 **teaspoon dried thyme**
2 **whole bay leaves**
1 **pork roast (about 4 pounds)**
Olive oil
2 **cups green grapes**
1 **cup dried apricots**
1 **cup dried prunes**
2 **cloves garlic, minced**
1 **cup red wine**
Juice of ½ lemon

1. Combine water, salt, sugar, thyme and bay leaves in large resealable plastic food storage bag, or in plastic or glass container (do not use metal container). Add pork roast. Marinate overnight or up to 2 days in refrigerator, turning occasionally.

2. Remove roast from brine and lightly pat dry. Heat oil in skillet over medium heat until hot. Brown pork roast on all sides, cooking 5 to 10 minutes, turning as it browns. Transfer to **CROCK-POT®** slow cooker.

3. Add remaining ingredients. Stir gently to combine. Cover; cook on LOW 7 to 9 hours or on HIGH 3 to 5 hours.

Makes 6 to 8 servings

Fall-Apart Pork Roast with Mole

⅔ **cup whole almonds**
⅔ **cup raisins**
3 **tablespoons vegetable oil, divided**
½ **cup chopped onion**
4 **cloves garlic, chopped**
2¾ **pounds lean boneless pork shoulder roast, well trimmed**
1 **can (14½ ounces) diced fire-roasted tomatoes or diced tomatoes, undrained**
1 **cup cubed bread, any variety**
½ **cup chicken broth**
2 **ounces Mexican chocolate, chopped**
2 **tablespoons chipotle peppers in adobo sauce, chopped**
1 **teaspoon salt**
Fresh cilantro, coarsely chopped (optional)

1. Heat large skillet over medium-high heat until hot. Add almonds and toast 3 to 4 minutes, stirring frequently, until fragrant. Add raisins. Cook 1 to 2 minutes longer, stirring constantly, until raisins begin to plump. Place half of almond mixture in large mixing bowl. Reserve remaining half for garnish.

2. In same skillet, heat 1 tablespoon oil. Add onion and garlic. Cook and stir 2 to 3 minutes until softened. Add to almond mixture; set aside.

3. Heat remaining oil in same skillet. Add pork roast and brown on all sides, about 5 to 7 minutes. Transfer to **CROCK-POT®** slow cooker.

4. Combine tomatoes with juice, bread, broth, chocolate, chipotle peppers and salt with almond mixture. Purée mixture in blender, in 2 to 3 batches, until smooth. Pour purée over pork roast in **CROCK-POT®** slow cooker. Cover; cook on LOW 7 to 8 hours or on HIGH 3 to 4 hours or until pork is done.

5. Remove pork roast from **CROCK-POT®** slow cooker. Whisk sauce until smooth before spooning over pork roast. Garnish with reserved almond mixture and chopped cilantro, if desired.

Makes 6 servings

Boneless Pork Roast with Garlic

1 **boneless pork rib roast (2 to 2½ pounds), rinsed and patted dry**
  Salt and black pepper, to taste
3 **tablespoons olive oil, divided**
4 **cloves garlic, minced**
4 **tablespoons chopped fresh rosemary**
½ **lemon, cut into ⅛- to ¼-inch slices**
¼ **cup white wine**
½ **cup chicken stock**

1. Unroll the pork roast and season with salt and pepper. Combine 2 tablespoons oil, garlic and rosemary in small bowl. Rub over pork.

2. Roll and tie pork snugly with twine. Tuck lemon slices under twine and into ends of roast.

3. Heat remaining 1 tablespoon oil in skillet over medium heat until hot. Sear pork on all sides until just browned. Transfer to **CROCK-POT®** slow cooker.

4. Return skillet to heat. Add white wine and stock, stirring with wooden spoon to loosen any caramelized bits. Pour over pork. Cover; cook on LOW 8 to 9 hours or on HIGH 3½ to 4 hours.

5. Transfer roast to cutting board. Allow to rest for 10 minutes before removing twine and slicing. Adjust seasonings, if desired. To serve, pour pan juices over sliced pork.

Makes 4 to 6 servings

Heavenly Harvest Pork Roast

¼ cup pomegranate juice
¼ cup sugar
1 tablespoon salt
1 tablespoon garlic salt
1 tablespoon steak seasoning
1 teaspoon black pepper
1 pork roast, any type (4 to 5 pounds)
2 pears, cored, peeled and sliced thick
½ orange with peel, sliced thick

1. Combine pomegranate juice and sugar in small saucepan. Cook over low heat, stirring until sugar dissolves, about 2 minutes. Pour into **CROCK-POT®** slow cooker.

2. Blend salt, garlic salt, steak seasoning and pepper in small mixing bowl. Rub mixture over roast. Place roast in **CROCK-POT®** slow cooker. Turn roast to cover with juice mixture.

3. Top roast with pear and orange slices. Cover; cook on HIGH 6 to 8 hours or until tender. Serve with juice and fruit slices.

Makes 6 to 8 servings

Best Asian-Style Ribs

- **2 full racks baby back pork ribs, split into 3 sections each**
- **6 ounces hoisin sauce**
- **2 tablespoons minced fresh ginger**
- **½ cup maraschino cherries**
- **½ cup rice wine vinegar**
  Water to cover
- **4 green onions, chopped (optional)**

Combine ribs, hoisin sauce, ginger, cherries, vinegar and water in **CROCK-POT®** slow cooker. Cover; cook on LOW 6 to 7 hours or on HIGH 3 to 3½ hours or until pork is done. Sprinkle with green onions before serving, if desired.

Makes 6 to 8 servings

Golden Pork with Cinnamon-Sugar Apples

- **1 pork sirloin roast (about 3 pounds)**
- **1 can condensed golden mushroom soup, undiluted**
- **½ cup water**
- **¼ cup packed brown sugar**
- **2 tablespoons soy sauce**
- **¼ cup granulated sugar**
- **3 tablespoons ground cinnamon**
- **2 Granny Smith apples, cored and sliced**
  Hot cooked rice or noodles

1. Place pork in **CROCK-POT®** slow cooker.

2. Combine soup, water, brown sugar and soy sauce in medium bowl; stir to mix well. Pour over pork. Cover; cook on LOW 8 hours.

3. About 1 hour before serving, combine granulated sugar and cinnamon in medium resealable plastic food storage bag. Add apples; shake to coat well. Place apples on top of pork. Cover; cook 1 hour longer. Serve with rice or noodles.

Makes 6 servings

Best Asian-Style Ribs

Pork Chops à l'Orange

- **2 tablespoons extra-virgin olive oil**
- **8 pork chops**
- **⅓ cup orange juice**
- **2 tablespoons clover honey**
- **1 teaspoon salt**
- **1 teaspoon packed brown sugar**
- **1 teaspoon grated orange peel**
- **2 tablespoons cornstarch**
- **¼ cup water**

1. Heat oil in large skillet over medium-high heat until hot. Working in batches, sear chops on both sides, about 1 to 2 minutes, turning each chop as it browns; set aside.

2. Combine orange juice, honey, salt, brown sugar and orange peel in **CROCK-POT®** slow cooker. Add chops, turning each chop to coat well. Cover; cook on LOW 6 to 8 hours.

3. Transfer chops to warm plate. Pour cooking liquid into small heavy saucepan. Cook over medium-high heat until liquid begins to boil. Meanwhile, combine cornstarch and water in small bowl. Add to orange sauce. Stir well to combine. Reduce heat and simmer 5 minutes, or until thickened. Spoon sauce over chops, and serve immediately.

Makes 8 servings

Mango Ginger Pork Roast

- **1 pork shoulder roast (about 4 pounds)**
- **½ to 1 teaspoon ground ginger, or to taste**
  Salt and black pepper, to taste
- **2 cups mango salsa**
- **2 tablespoons honey**
- **¼ cup apricot preserves**
  Hot cooked rice

1. Season roast with ginger, salt and pepper. Transfer to **CROCK-POT®** slow cooker.

2. Combine salsa, honey and preserves. Pour over roast. Cover; cook on LOW 6 to 8 hours. Turn **CROCK-POT®** slow cooker to HIGH and cook 3 to 4 hours longer, or until roast is tender. Serve with rice.

Makes 4 to 6 servings

Backroads Ham and Potato Casserole

- **2 pounds baking potatoes, cut into 1-inch cubes**
- **½ teaspoon dried thyme**
- **12 ounces cubed ham**
- **1 can (10¾ ounces) condensed cream of chicken soup, undiluted**
- **4 ounces cream cheese, cut into ½-inch cubes**
- **½ cup finely chopped green onions**
- **½ cup frozen green peas, thawed**

1. Coat **CROCK-POT®** slow cooker with nonstick cooking spray. Place potatoes in bottom. Add thyme and ham. Spread soup evenly over potatoes and ham. Cover; cook on HIGH 3 to 5 hours.

2. Gently stir in cream cheese, green onions and peas. Cover; cook 5 minutes longer or until cheese is melted.

Makes 4 to 6 servings

Mango Ginger Pork Roast

Sweet & Spicy Pork Picadillo

1 tablespoon olive oil
1 yellow onion, cut into ¼-inch dice
2 cloves garlic, minced
1 pound boneless pork country-style ribs, trimmed of excess fat and cut into 1-inch cubes
1 can (14½ ounces) diced tomatoes, undrained
3 tablespoons cider vinegar
2 chipotle peppers (canned, in adobo), chopped*
½ cup raisins, chopped
½ teaspoon cumin
½ teaspoon ground cinnamon
Salt and black pepper, to taste

*If using dried chipotles, soak in warm water to soften before chopping—about 20 minutes.

1. Heat oil in skillet over medium-low heat until hot. Cook and stir onions and garlic until translucent, about 4 minutes.

2. Add pork to skillet and brown. Transfer to **CROCK-POT®** slow cooker.

3. Combine tomatoes with juice, vinegar, chipotle peppers, raisins, cumin and cinnamon in medium bowl. Pour over pork. Cover; cook on LOW 5 hours or on HIGH 3 hours, or until pork is fork-tender. Shred pork using 2 forks. Cook 30 minutes longer. Adjust seasonings before serving, if desired.

Makes 4 servings

Barbecue Ribs

Canola oil or vegetable oil
2 small red onions, finely chopped
3 to 4 cloves garlic, minced
1 cup ketchup
1 cup packed brown sugar
½ cup cider vinegar
Juice of 1 lemon
2 tablespoons Worcestershire sauce
1 tablespoon hot pepper sauce, or to taste
½ teaspoon chili powder
2 racks pork baby back ribs, cut into 3- to 4-rib sections

1. Heat oil in skillet over medium heat until hot. Add onions and garlic. Cook and stir until softened and lightly browned. Stir in ketchup, brown sugar, vinegar, lemon juice, Worcestershire sauce, hot sauce and chili powder. Simmer gently about 5 minutes. Remove half of sauce and reserve.

2. Transfer remaining sauce to **CROCK-POT®** slow cooker. Add ribs, stirring to coat. Cover; cook on LOW 7 to 9 hours or on HIGH 4 to 6 hours. To serve, cut ribs between bones and pass reserved sauce.

Makes 6 servings

Italian Sausage and Peppers

- **3 cups bell pepper chunks (1 inch), preferably a mix of red, yellow and green**
- **1 small onion, cut into thin wedges**
- **3 cloves garlic, minced**
- **4 links hot or mild Italian sausage (about 1 pound)**
- **1 cup marinara or pasta sauce**
- **¼ cup red wine or port**
- **1 tablespoon cornstarch**
- **1 tablespoon water**
- **Hot cooked spaghetti**
- **¼ cup grated Parmesan or Romano cheese**

1. Coat **CROCK-POT®** slow cooker with nonstick cooking spray. Add bell peppers, onion and garlic. Arrange sausage over vegetables.

2. Combine pasta sauce and wine; pour over sausage. Cover; cook on LOW 8 to 9 hours or on HIGH 4 to 5 hours, or until sausage is cooked through and vegetables are very tender.

3. Transfer sausage to serving platter; cover with foil to keep warm. Skim off and discard fat from cooking liquid.

4. Turn heat to HIGH. Mix cornstarch with water until smooth; add to **CROCK-POT®** slow cooker. Cook 15 minutes or until sauce has thickened, stirring once. Serve sauce over spaghetti and sausage; top with cheese.

Makes 4 servings

Scalloped Potatoes and Ham

6 large russet potatoes, sliced into ¼-inch rounds
1 ham steak (about 1½ pounds), cut into cubes
1 can (10¾ ounces) condensed cream of mushroom soup, undiluted
1 soup can water
1 cup (about 4 ounces) shredded Cheddar cheese
Grill seasoning, to taste

1. Coat **CROCK-POT®** slow cooker with nonstick cooking spray. Arrange potatoes and ham in layers in **CROCK-POT®** slow cooker.

2. Combine soup, water, cheese and grill seasoning in large glass measure; pour over potatoes and ham. Cover; cook on HIGH about 3½ hours or until potatoes are fork-tender. Turn heat to LOW and continue cooking about 1 hour more.

Makes 5 to 6 servings

SIDE DISHES

Slow Cooking Side Dishes

Preparing vegetables

Vegetables, especially root vegetables, can take longer to cook than meats. Cut vegetables into uniform pieces so they finish cooking at the same time. Root vegetables—such as potatoes, carrots, and turnips—should be cut into small pieces and placed on the bottom of the slow cooker so they are always in liquid. Vegetables should not be precooked. Occasionally a recipe will call for sautéing onions and garlic; this is usually done to reduce their sharpness. For example, in Classic French Onion Soup *(page 122)*, the onions are sautéed for 15 minutes to allow them to develop a caramelized flavor, which adds a very distinctive note to the finished soup.

You may choose to add strong-flavored vegetables such as broccoli, cabbage, and cauliflower during the last hour or two of cooking. Shorter cooking prevents their flavor from overwhelming the dish. Tender, delicate vegetables, such as spinach, green onions, and snow peas, should also be added during the last hour of cooking to prevent overcooking them.

Rice

Choose long-grain converted rice (or Arborio rice when suggested) or wild

You Don't Know Beans?

It's so simple to save money preparing dried beans instead of using canned.

It's best to presoak dried beans before cooking them in a slow cooker. This softens them and gives them a head start on cooking. Softening beans reduces the cooking time. (Lentils and split peas do not need to be softened.) The two methods for presoaking follow:

Traditional method

Place dried beans that have been sorted and rinsed in a bowl. Cover them with cold unsalted water and let them stand overnight. Drain off the water and place the beans in the slow cooker.

Quick method

Place sorted and rinsed dried beans in a medium or large saucepan; cover them with twice their volume of cold unsalted water. Bring the water to a boil over high heat. Boil for 2 minutes. Remove the saucepan from the heat, cover it and let it stand for 1 hour. Drain off the water and place the beans in the slow cooker.

Even when beans are presoaked they take a long time to cook. Avoid adding acids or sweeteners to the beans until they are soft. Acids and sweeteners will slow down the softening process and will lengthen the cooking process. Acids include tomatoes, vinegar, and citrus juices; sweeteners include sugar, honey, and molasses. Add these items toward the end of the cooking time.

rice for best results. Extended slow cooking can turn other types of rice into mush; if you prefer other types of rice, cook them conventionally and add them to the slow cooker during the last 15 minutes of cooking. You can add a small amount (½ cup) of uncooked rice to the slow cooker soup or other dish; be sure to add it to boiling liquid during the last hour of cooking.

If you wish to add rice to a recipe that doesn't include it, you will need to adjust the liquid as well. Add an equal amount of water or broth before you add the rice.

Pasta

Pasta needs to be cooked in a large quantity of boiling water; it should not be cooked in a slow cooker. However, you can add small amounts ($\frac{1}{2}$ to 1 cup) of small pasta—such as orzo, small shell macaroni, ditali, and short lengths of linguine—to boiling liquid during the last one hour of slow cooking. You may also cook pasta in boiling water and add it to the slow cooker during the last 30 minutes of cooking.

RICE & PASTA

Artichoke and Tomato Paella

4 cups vegetable broth

2 cups converted white rice

½ package (10-ounce size) frozen chopped spinach, thawed and drained

1 green bell pepper, cored, seeded and chopped

1 medium ripe tomato, sliced into wedges

1 medium yellow onion, chopped

1 medium carrot, peeled and diced

3 cloves garlic, minced

1 tablespoon minced flat-leaf parsley

1 teaspoon salt

½ teaspoon black pepper

1 can (13¾ ounces) artichoke hearts, quartered, rinsed and well-drained

½ cup frozen peas

1. Combine broth, rice, spinach, bell pepper, tomato, onion, carrot, garlic, parsley, salt and pepper in **CROCK-POT®** slow cooker. Mix thoroughly. Cover; cook on LOW 4 hours or on HIGH 2 hours.

2. Before serving, add artichoke hearts and peas. Cover; cook on HIGH 15 minutes. Mix well before serving.

Makes 8 servings

Creamy Chicken and Spinach Lasagna

- 1¼ cups shredded Swiss or mozzarella cheese, divided
- 1 cup ricotta cheese
- 1 teaspoon dried oregano
- ¼ teaspoon red pepper flakes
- 1 container (10 ounces) refrigerated Alfredo pasta sauce
- ⅓ cup water
- 4 no-boil lasagna noodles
- 1 package (10 ounces) frozen chopped spinach, thawed and squeezed dry
- 1½ cups cooked diced chicken
- ¼ cup grated Parmesan cheese
  Red pepper flakes, for garnish

1. Combine 1 cup Swiss cheese, ricotta, oregano and red pepper flakes in small bowl; set aside. Blend Alfredo sauce with water; set aside.

2. Coat **CROCK-POT®** slow cooker with nonstick cooking spray. Break 2 lasagna noodles in half and place on bottom. Spread half of ricotta mixture over noodles. Top with half of spinach. Arrange half of chicken and half of Parmesan over spinach. Pour half of Alfredo mixture over top. Repeat layers, beginning with noodles and ending with Alfredo mixture. Cover; cook on LOW 3 hours.

3. Sprinkle remaining ¼ cup Swiss cheese on top. Cover and let stand 5 minutes or until cheese is melted. To serve, cut into squares or wedges. Garnish with pepper flakes, if desired.

Makes 4 servings

Wild Rice with Fruit & Nuts

- **2 cups wild rice (or wild rice blend), rinsed***
- **½ cup dried cranberries**
- **½ cup chopped raisins**
- **½ cup chopped dried apricots**
- **½ cup almond slivers, toasted****
- **5 to 6 cups chicken broth**
- **1 cup orange juice**
- **2 tablespoons butter, melted**
- **1 teaspoon ground cumin**
- **2 green onions, thinly sliced**
- **2 to 3 tablespoons chopped fresh parsley**
- **Salt and black pepper, to taste**

Do not use parboiled rice or a blend containing parboiled rice.

**To toast almonds, spread in single layer in heavy-bottomed skillet. Cook over medium heat 1 to 2 minutes, stirring frequently, until nuts are lightly browned. Remove from skillet immediately. Cool before using.*

1. Combine wild rice, cranberries, raisins, apricots and almonds in **CROCK-POT®** slow cooker.

2. Combine broth, orange juice, butter and cumin in medium bowl. Pour mixture over rice and stir to mix.

3. Cover; cook on LOW 7 hours or on HIGH 2½ to 3 hours. Stir once, adding more hot broth if necessary.

4. When rice is soft, add green onions and parsley. Adjust seasonings, if desired. Cook 10 minutes longer and serve.

Makes 6 to 8 servings

Asiago and Asparagus Risotto-Style Rice

- 2 **cups chopped onion**
- 1 **cup uncooked converted rice**
- 2 **medium cloves garlic, minced**
- 1 **can (14½ ounces) chicken broth**
- ½ **pound asparagus spears, trimmed and broken into 1-inch pieces**
- 1 **to 1¼ cups half-and-half, divided**
- ½ **cup (about 4 ounces) shredded Asiago cheese, plus more for garnish**
- ¼ **cup (½ stick) butter, cut into small pieces**
- 2 **ounces pine nuts or slivered almonds, toasted**
- 1 **teaspoon salt**

1. Combine onion, rice, garlic and broth in **CROCK-POT®** slow cooker. Stir until well blended; cover and cook 2 hours on HIGH or until rice is done.

2. Stir in asparagus and ½ cup half-and-half. Cover and cook 20 to 30 minutes more or until asparagus is just tender.

3. Stir in remaining ingredients, then cover and let stand 5 minutes to allow cheese to melt slightly. Fluff with fork and garnish with additional Asiago cheese, if desired, before serving.

Makes 4 servings

Tip

Risotto is a classic creamy rice dish of northern Italy. It can be made with a wide variety of ingredients; fresh vegetables and cheeses such as Asiago work especially well in risottos. Parmesan cheese, shellfish, white wine and herbs are also popular additions.

Pesto Rice and Beans

- 1 **can (15 ounces) Great Northern beans, rinsed and drained**
- 1 **can (14 ounces) chicken broth**
- ¾ **cup uncooked converted long-grain rice**
- 1½ **cups frozen cut green beans, thawed and drained**
- ½ **cup prepared pesto**
  Grated Parmesan cheese (optional)

1. Combine beans, broth and rice in **CROCK-POT®** slow cooker. Cover; cook on LOW 2 hours.

2. Stir in green beans. Cover; cook 1 hour or until rice and beans are tender.

3. Turn off **CROCK-POT®** slow cooker and transfer stoneware to heatproof surface. Stir in pesto and Parmesan cheese, if desired. Let stand, covered, 5 minutes or until cheese is melted. Serve immediately.

Makes 8 servings

Tip

*Choose converted long-grain rice (or Arborio rice when suggested) or wild rice for best results. Long, slow cooking can turn other types of rice into mush; if you prefer to use another type of rice instead of converted rice, cook it on the stove-top and add it to the **CROCK-POT®** slow cooker during the last 15 minutes of cooking.*

Turkey Vegetable Chili Mac

¾ **pound ground turkey breast**
1 **can (about 15 ounces) black beans, rinsed and drained**
1 **can (about 14 ounces) Mexican-style diced tomatoes**
1 **can (about 14 ounces) no-salt-added diced tomatoes**
1 **cup frozen corn**
½ **cup chopped onion**
2 **cloves garlic, minced**
1 **teaspoon Mexican seasoning**
½ **cup (about 2 ounces) uncooked elbow macaroni**
⅓ **cup sour cream**

1. Lightly coat large nonstick skillet with nonstick cooking spray. Add turkey; cook until browned. Transfer to **CROCK-POT®** slow cooker. Add beans, tomatoes, corn, onion, garlic and seasoning. Cover; cook on LOW 4 to 5 hours.

2. Stir in macaroni. Cover; cook 10 minutes. Stir. Cover; cook 20 to 30 minutes or until pasta is tender. Serve with sour cream.

Makes 6 servings

Tip

Feel free to substitute 2 ounces of any other pasta. Short pasta shapes like cavatappi, penne or rigatoni (which are sometimes called "cut pastas" because they are cut into pieces during the manufacturing process) can be added straight out of the packages. Longer shapes such as linguine, fettuccine or spaghetti should be broken in halves or thirds before being stirred in so that all the pasta can be fully immersed in the sauce.

No-Fuss Macaroni & Cheese

- 2 cups (about 8 ounces) uncooked elbow macaroni
- 4 ounces light pasteurized processed cheese, cubed
- 1 cup (4 ounces) shredded mild Cheddar cheese
- ½ teaspoon salt
- ⅛ teaspoon black pepper
- 1½ cups fat-free (skim) milk

Combine macaroni, cheeses, salt and pepper in **CROCK-POT®** slow cooker. Pour milk over all. Cover; cook on LOW 2 to 3 hours, stirring after 20 to 30 minutes.

Makes 6 to 8 servings

Easy Dirty Rice

½ **pound bulk Italian sausage**
2 **cups water**
1 **cup uncooked long-grain rice**
1 **large onion, finely chopped**
1 **large green bell pepper, finely chopped**
½ **cup finely chopped celery**
1½ **teaspoons salt**
½ **teaspoon ground red pepper**
½ **cup chopped fresh parsley**

1. Brown sausage in skillet 6 to 8 minutes over medium-high heat, stirring to break up meat. Drain fat. Place sausage in **CROCK-POT®** slow cooker.

2. Stir in all remaining ingredients except parsley. Cover; cook on LOW 2 hours. Stir in parsley.

Makes 4 servings

Arroz con Queso

- 1 **can (16 ounces) whole tomatoes, crushed**
- 1 **can (15 ounces) black beans, rinsed and drained**
- 1½ **cups uncooked converted long-grain rice**
- 1 **onion, chopped**
- 1 **cup cottage cheese**
- 1 **can (4 ounces) chopped green chilies**
- 2 **tablespoons vegetable oil**
- 3 **teaspoons minced garlic**
- 2 **cups grated Monterey Jack cheese, divided**

Combine tomatoes, beans, rice, onion, cottage cheese, chilies, oil, garlic and 1 cup cheese in **CROCK-POT®** slow cooker; mix thoroughly. Cover; cook on LOW 6 to 9 hours or until liquid is absorbed. Sprinkle with remaining cheese before serving.

Makes 8 to 10 servings

Southwestern Mac and Cheese

1 package (8 ounces) elbow macaroni, uncooked

1 can (about 14 ounces) diced tomatoes with green peppers and onions, undrained

1 can (10 ounces) diced tomatoes with green chilies, undrained

1½ cups salsa

3 cups (about 12 ounces) shredded Mexican cheese blend, divided

1. Lightly coat inside of **CROCK-POT®** slow cooker with nonstick cooking spray. Stir together macaroni, tomatoes and their juices, salsa and 2 cups cheese in prepared **CROCK-POT®** slow cooker. Cover and cook on LOW 3 hours and 45 minutes or until macaroni is tender.

2. Sprinkle remaining 1 cup cheese over contents of **CROCK-POT®** slow cooker. Cover and cook 15 minutes more or until cheese on top melts.

Makes 6 servings

South-of-the-Border Macaroni & Cheese

- **5 cups cooked rotini pasta**
- **2 cups (8 ounces) cubed American cheese**
- **1 can (12 ounces) evaporated milk**
- **1 cup (4 ounces) cubed sharp Cheddar cheese**
- **1 can (4 ounces) diced green chiles, drained**
- **2 teaspoons chili powder**
- **2 medium tomatoes, seeded and chopped**
- **5 green onions, sliced**

1. Combine pasta, American cheese, evaporated milk, Cheddar cheese, chiles and chili powder in **CROCK-POT®** slow cooker; mix well. Cover; cook on HIGH 2 hours, stirring occasionally.

2. Stir in tomatoes and green onions; continue cooking until heated through.

Makes 4 servings

Spanish Paella-Style Rice

2 cans (14½ ounces each) chicken broth
1½ cups uncooked converted long-grain rice
1 small red bell pepper, diced
⅓ cup dry white wine or water
½ teaspoon saffron threads, crushed or ½ teaspoon ground turmeric
⅛ teaspoon red pepper flakes
½ cup frozen peas, thawed
Salt, to taste

1. Combine broth, rice, bell pepper, wine, saffron and red pepper flakes in **CROCK-POT®** slow cooker; mix well. Cover; cook on LOW 4 hours or until liquid is absorbed.

2. Stir in peas. Cover; cook 15 to 30 minutes or until peas are hot. Season with salt.

Makes 6 servings

Tip
Paella can contain a variety of meats as well. For more authenticity — and to turn this dish into a delicious main course — add ½ cup cooked ham, chicken, chorizo or seafood when you add the peas.

VEGETABLES

Herbed Fall Vegetables

- **2 medium Yukon Gold potatoes, peeled and cut into ½-inch dice**
- **2 medium sweet potatoes, peeled and cut into ½-inch dice**
- **3 parsnips, peeled and cut into ½-inch dice**
- **1 medium head of fennel, sliced and cut into ½-inch dice**
- **½ to ¾ cup chopped fresh herbs, such as tarragon, parsley, sage or thyme**
- **¼ cup (½ stick) butter, cut into small pieces**
- **1 cup chicken broth**
- **1 tablespoon Dijon mustard**
- **1 tablespoon salt**
  Freshly ground black pepper, to taste

1. Combine potatoes, parsnips, fennel, herbs and butter in **CROCK-POT®** slow cooker.

2. Whisk together broth, mustard, salt and pepper in small bowl. Pour mixture over vegetables. Cover; cook on LOW 4½ hours or on HIGH 3 hours or until vegetables are tender, stirring occasionally to ensure even cooking.

Makes 6 servings

Cheesy Broccoli Casserole

2 **packages (10 ounces each) frozen chopped broccoli, thawed**

1 **can (10¾ ounces) condensed cream of celery soup, undiluted**

1¼ **cups shredded sharp Cheddar cheese, divided**

¼ **cup minced onion**

½ **teaspoon celery seed**

1 **teaspoon paprika**

1 **teaspoon hot pepper sauce**

1 **cup crushed potato chips or saltine crackers**

1. Coat **CROCK-POT®** slow cooker with nonstick cooking spray. Combine broccoli, soup, 1 cup cheese, onion, celery seed, paprika and hot sauce in **CROCK-POT®** slow cooker; mix well. Cover; cook on LOW 5 to 6 hours or on HIGH 2½ to 3 hours, or until done.

2. Uncover; sprinkle top with potato chips and remaining ¼ cup cheese. Cook, uncovered, on LOW 30 to 60 minutes or on HIGH 15 to 30 minutes, or until cheese melts.

Makes 4 to 6 servings

Tip

For a change in taste, prepare with thawed chopped spinach instead of broccoli, and top with crushed crackers or spicy croutons to complement the cheesy crust.

Lemon-Mint Red Potatoes

- 2 **pounds new red potatoes**
- 3 **tablespoons extra-virgin olive oil**
- ¾ **teaspoon dried Greek seasoning or dried oregano leaves**
- ¼ **teaspoon garlic powder**
- 1 **teaspoon salt**
- ¼ **teaspoon black pepper**
- 2 **tablespoons lemon juice**
- 1 **teaspoon grated lemon peel**
- 2 **tablespoons butter**
- ¼ **cup chopped fresh mint leaves, divided**

1. Coat inside of **CROCK-POT**® slow cooker with nonstick cooking spray. Add potatoes and oil, stirring gently to coat. Sprinkle with Greek seasoning, garlic powder, salt and pepper. Cover and cook on LOW 7 hours or on HIGH 4 hours.

2. Stir in lemon juice, lemon peel, butter and 2 tablespoons mint. Stir until butter is completely melted. Cover and cook 15 minutes to allow flavors to blend. Sprinkle with remaining mint.

Makes 4 servings

Tip

It's easy to prepare this recipe ahead of time; simply follow instructions as listed and then turn off heat and let stand at room temperature for up to 2 hours. Reheat or serve at room temperature.

Supper Squash Medley

- **2 butternut squash, peeled, seeded and diced**
- **1 can (28 ounces) tomatoes, undrained**
- **1 can (15 ounces) corn, drained**
- **2 onions, chopped**
- **2 green bell peppers, chopped**
- **2 teaspoons minced garlic**
- **2 green chiles, chopped**
- **1 cup chicken broth**
- **1 teaspoon salt**
- **½ teaspoon black pepper**
- **1 can (6 ounces) tomato paste**

1. Combine squash, tomatoes with juice, corn, onions, bell peppers, garlic, chiles, broth, salt and pepper in **CROCK-POT®** slow cooker. Cover; cook on LOW 6 hours.

2. Remove about ½ cup cooking liquid and blend with tomato paste. Add back to **CROCK-POT®** slow cooker and stir well. Cook 30 minutes or until mixture is slightly thickened and heated through.

Makes 8 to 10 servings

Orange-Spiced Sweet Potatoes

- 2 pounds sweet potatoes, peeled and diced
- ½ cup packed dark brown sugar
- ½ cup (1 stick) butter, cut into small pieces
- 1 teaspoon ground cinnamon
- ½ teaspoon ground nutmeg
- ½ teaspoon grated orange peel
- Juice of 1 medium orange
- ¼ teaspoon salt
- 1 teaspoon vanilla
- Chopped toasted pecans (optional)

Place all ingredients except pecans in **CROCK-POT®** slow cooker. Cover; cook on LOW 4 hours or on HIGH 2 hours or until potatoes are tender. Sprinkle with pecans before serving, if desired.

Makes 8 servings

Tip

For a creamy variation, mash potatoes with a hand masher or electric mixer, and add ¼ cup milk or whipping cream for moist consistency. Sprinkle with cinnamon-sugar, and sprinkle on toasted pecans, if desired.

Bacon and Cheese Brunch Potatoes

3 medium russet potatoes (about 2 pounds), peeled and cut into 1-inch dice
1 cup chopped onion
½ teaspoon seasoned salt
4 slices crisply cooked bacon, crumbled
1 cup (4 ounces) shredded sharp Cheddar cheese
1 tablespoon water or chicken broth

1. Coat **CROCK-POT®** slow cooker with cooking spray. Place half of potatoes in **CROCK-POT®** slow cooker. Sprinkle ½ of onion and seasoned salt over potatoes; top with ½ of bacon and cheese. Repeat layers, ending with cheese. Sprinkle water over top.

2. Cover; cook on LOW 6 hours or on HIGH 3½ hours, or until potatoes and onion are tender. Stir gently to mix and serve hot.

Makes 6 servings

Creamy Curried Spinach

- **3 packages (10 ounces each) frozen spinach, thawed**
- **1 onion, chopped**
- **4 teaspoons minced garlic**
- **2 tablespoons curry powder**
- **2 tablespoons butter, melted**
- **¼ cup chicken broth**
- **¼ cup heavy cream**
- **1 teaspoon lemon juice**

Combine spinach, onion, garlic, curry powder, butter and broth in **CROCK-POT®** slow cooker. Cover; cook on LOW 3 to 4 hours or on HIGH 2 hours or until done. Stir in cream and lemon juice 30 minutes before end of cooking time.

Makes 6 to 8 servings

Lemon and Tangerine Glazed Carrots

- **6 cups sliced carrots**
- **1½ cups apple juice**
- **6 tablespoons butter**
- **¼ cup packed brown sugar**
- **2 tablespoons grated lemon peel**
- **2 tablespoons grated tangerine peel**
- **½ teaspoon salt**
- **Fresh parsley, chopped (optional)**

Combine all ingredients in **CROCK-POT®** slow cooker. Cover; cook on LOW 4 to 5 hours or on HIGH 1 to 3 hours. Garnish with chopped parsley, if desired.

Makes 10 to 12 servings

Gratin Potatoes with Asiago Cheese

6 slices bacon, cut into 1-inch pieces
6 medium baking potatoes, peeled and thinly sliced
½ cup grated Asiago cheese
Salt and black pepper, to taste
1½ cups heavy cream

1. Heat skillet over medium heat until hot. Add bacon. Cook and stir until crispy. Transfer to paper towel-lined plate with slotted spoon to drain.

2. Pour bacon fat from skillet into **CROCK-POT®** slow cooker. Layer one fourth of potatoes on bottom of **CROCK-POT®** slow cooker. Sprinkle one fourth of bacon over potatoes and top with one fourth of cheese. Add salt and pepper. Repeat layers. Pour cream over all. Cover; cook on LOW 7 to 9 hours or on HIGH 5 to 6 hours. Adjust salt and pepper, if desired.

Makes 4 to 6 servings

Winter Squash and Apples

1	teaspoon salt
½	teaspoon black pepper
1	butternut squash (about 2 pounds), peeled and seeded
2	apples, cored and cut into slices
1	medium onion, quartered and sliced
1½	tablespoons butter

1. Combine salt and pepper in small bowl; set aside.

2. Cut squash into 2-inch pieces; place in **CROCK-POT**® slow cooker. Add apples and onion. Sprinkle with salt mixture; stir well. Cover; cook on LOW 6 to 7 hours or until vegetables are tender.

3. Just before serving, stir in butter and season to taste with additional salt and pepper.

Makes 4 to 6 servings

Red Cabbage and Apples

1 **small head red cabbage, cored and thinly sliced**
3 **medium apples, peeled and grated**
¾ **cup sugar**
½ **cup red wine vinegar**
1 **teaspoon ground cloves**
1 **cup crisp-cooked and crumbled bacon (optional)**
Fresh apple slices (optional)

Combine cabbage, apples, sugar, vinegar and cloves in **CROCK-POT**® slow cooker. Cover; cook on HIGH 6 hours, stirring after 3 hours. To serve, sprinkle with bacon and garnish with apple slices, if desired.

Makes 4 to 6 servings

Boston Baked Beans

2 **pounds small dry white beans**
12 **cups water**
   Olive oil
¼ **cup finely chopped salt pork or thick-sliced bacon**
1 **cup molasses**
½ **cup chopped onions**
½ **cup packed dark brown sugar**
2 **tablespoons dry mustard**
2 **teaspoons salt**

1. Soak beans in water in uncovered **CROCK-POT®** slow cooker overnight (or a minimum of 8 hours). After soaking, cover; cook on LOW 3 hours. Drain liquid, reserving 1 cup. Remove beans; set aside.

2. Heat oil in skillet over medium heat until hot. Add salt pork. Cook and stir 5 to 10 minutes to render fat. Remove with slotted spoon and drain on paper towels. Transfer to **CROCK-POT®** slow cooker.

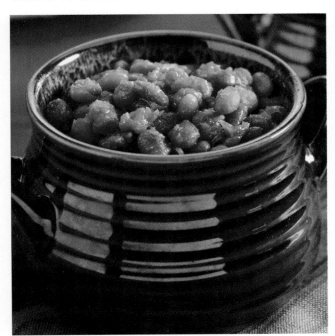

3. Add reserved 1 cup cooking liquid, beans, and remaining ingredients; stir well to combine. Cover; cook on LOW 10 to 12 hours or on HIGH 6 to 8 hours.

Makes 8 servings

SOUPS & STEWS

Slow Cooking Soups & Stews

Serving soup and stew

Few recipes are as well suited for slow cooking as soups and stews. They take full advantage of the magic of braising to turn inexpensive cuts of meat and root vegetables into hearty, satisfying fare.

The one drawback to using inexpensive cuts of meat in slow cooking is that they frequently contain hidden quantities of fat that renders out during cooking. If you have the time, the best way to remove and discard any unwanted fat is to refrigerate the soup overnight. The fat will float to the surface and congeal where it is easily spooned off and discarded.

Failing that, turn off the slow cooker and don't stir the soup for at least 15 minutes so as much fat floats to the surface as possible. Use a soup ladle to skim it off and discard it.

Thickening stews

Thickeners are usually added during the last 15 to 30 minutes of cooking. The amount of liquid created in a slow cooker dish may vary from unit to unit. Cooking on low heat often produces more juices than cooking on high. Removing the lid repeatedly during cooking will reduce liquids, but also adds to the cooking time by allowing heat to escape. If there doesn't seem to be much liquid, it is best to use only a reduced portion (one-half to three-fourths of the listed amount) of the thickening agent, adding more if necessary. If a dish becomes too thick, simply add additional broth or water to thin the sauce.

Flour: All-purpose flour is most often used in the recipes in this book. Place flour in a small bowl or cup and stir in enough cold water to make a thin, lump-free mixture; a whisk can help eliminate lumps. With the slow cooker on HIGH, quickly stir the flour mixture into the liquid in the slow cooker. Cook, stirring frequently, until the mixture thickens. Instant flour may be substituted; it can be stirred directly into hot liquid.

Cornstarch: Cornstarch gives sauces a clear, shiny appearance; it is used most often for sweet dessert sauces and stir-fry sauces. Place cornstarch in a small bowl or cup and stir in cold water, stirring until the cornstarch dissolves. Quickly stir this mixture into the liquid in the slow cooker; the sauce will thicken as soon as the liquid boils. Cornstarch breaks down with too much heat, so never add it at the beginning of the slow cooking process. And as soon as the sauce thickens, turn off the heat.

Arrowroot: Arrowroot (or arrowroot flour) is a ground powder of a tropical root; it produces a clear sauce. Those who are allergic to wheat often use it in place of flour. Place arrowroot in a small bowl or cup and stir in cold water until the mixture is smooth. Quickly stir this mixture into the liquid in the slow cooker. Unlike cornstarch, arrowroot thickens below the boiling point so it can thicken sauces easily with the low heat of a slow cooker. Too much stirring can break down an arrowroot mixture, so be sure and use it just before serving.

Tapioca: Tapioca is a starchy substance extracted from the root of the cassava plant. It comes in many forms; the quick-cooking form is used in several recipes in this book. Tapioca's greatest advantage is that it withstands long cooking, making it an ideal choice for slow cooking. Add it at the beginning of cooking and you'll get a clear thickened sauce in the finished dish. Dishes with tapioca as a thickener are best cooked on the low setting; tapioca may become stringy when boiled for a long time.

SOUPS

Hearty Chicken Noodle Soup

1¼ pounds boneless, skinless chicken breasts
1¼ pounds boneless, skinless chicken thighs
12 baby carrots, cut into ½-inch pieces
4 stalks celery, cut into ½-inch pieces
¾ cup finely chopped onion
1 teaspoon dried parsley flakes
½ teaspoon black pepper
¼ teaspoon ground red pepper
1 teaspoon salt
4 cans (14½ ounces each) chicken broth
4 chicken-flavored bouillon cubes
2 cups uncooked egg noodles

1. Cut chicken into bite-size pieces. Place in **CROCK-POT**® slow cooker. Add carrots, celery, onion, parsley, black pepper, red pepper, salt, chicken broth and bouillon cubes. Cover; cook on LOW 5 to 6 hours.

2. Stir in egg noodles. Turn temperature to HIGH. Cook 30 minutes longer or until noodles are tender.

Makes 8 to 10 servings

Chicken Tortilla Soup

- **4 boneless, skinless chicken thighs**
- **2 cans (15 ounces each) diced tomatoes, undrained**
- **1 can (4 ounces) chopped mild green chilies, drained**
- **½ to 1 cup chicken broth**
- **1 yellow onion, diced**
- **2 cloves garlic, minced**
- **1 teaspoon ground cumin**
  Salt and black pepper, to taste
- **4 corn tortillas, sliced into ¼-inch strips**
- **2 tablespoons chopped fresh cilantro**
- **½ cup shredded Monterey Jack cheese**
- **1 avocado, peeled, diced and tossed with lime juice**
  to prevent browning
  Lime wedges

1. Place chicken in **CROCK-POT®** slow cooker. Combine tomatoes with juice, chilies, ½ cup broth, onion, garlic and cumin in small bowl. Pour mixture over chicken.

2. Cover; cook on LOW 6 hours or on HIGH 3 hours, or until chicken is tender. Remove chicken from **CROCK-POT®** slow cooker. Shred with 2 forks. Return to cooking liquid. Adjust seasonings, adding salt and pepper and more broth, if necessary.

3. Just before serving, add tortillas and cilantro to **CROCK-POT®** slow cooker. Stir to blend. Serve in soup bowls, topping each serving with cheese, avocado and a squeeze of lime juice.

Makes 4 to 6 servings

Minestrone Alla Milanese

1 cup diced red potatoes
1 cup coarsely chopped carrots
2 cans (14½ ounces each) beef broth
1 can (14½ ounces) diced tomatoes, undrained
1 cup coarsely chopped green cabbage
1 cup sliced zucchini
¾ cup chopped onion
¾ cup sliced fresh green beans
¾ cup coarsely chopped celery
¾ cup water
2 tablespoons olive oil
1 clove garlic, minced
½ teaspoon dried basil
¼ teaspoon dried rosemary
1 bay leaf
1 can (15 ounces) cannellini beans, rinsed and drained
Shredded Parmesan cheese (optional)

1. Combine all ingredients except cannellini beans and cheese in **CROCK-POT®** slow cooker; mix well. Cover; cook on LOW 5 to 6 hours.

2. Add cannellini beans. Cover; cook on LOW 1 hour or until vegetables are tender.

3. Remove and discard bay leaf. Garnish with cheese, if desired.

Makes 8 to 10 servings

Northwoods Smoked Ham and Bean Soup

- 2 **tablespoons olive oil**
- 2 **large onions, chopped**
- 6 **cloves garlic, peeled and minced**
- 6 **cups chicken stock**
- 2 **smoked ham hocks**
- 2 **cups cubed cooked smoked ham**
- 1 **can (28 ounces) whole peeled plum tomatoes, drained and coarsely chopped**
- 1 **bunch fresh parsley, stemmed and chopped**
- 4 **sprigs fresh thyme**
- 4 **bay leaves**
- 2 **cans (15 ounces each) cannellini beans, drained and rinsed**
- ½ **pound cooked orecchiette, cavatelli or ditalini pasta**
  Kosher salt and black pepper

1. Heat olive oil in skillet over medium heat. Add onions and cook, stirring occasionally, until soft and fragrant, about 10 minutes. Add garlic and cook 1 minute.

2. Place onion and garlic mixture, stock, ham hocks, ham, tomatoes, parsley, thyme and bay leaves in **CROCK-POT®** slow cooker. Cook on LOW 10 hours or on HIGH 6 hours.

3. Stir in beans and pasta and continue to cook on HIGH until heated through.

4. Season to taste with salt and pepper and serve.

Makes 6 to 8 servings

Classic French Onion Soup

¼ **cup (½ stick) butter**
3 **large yellow onions, sliced**
1 **cup dry white wine**
3 **cans (14½ ounces each) beef or chicken broth**
1 **teaspoon Worcestershire sauce**
½ **teaspoon salt**
½ **teaspoon dried thyme leaves**
4 **slices French bread, toasted**
1 **cup (4 ounces) shredded Swiss cheese**
Fresh thyme (optional)

1. Melt butter in large skillet over medium heat. Add onions, cook and stir 15 minutes or until onions are soft and lightly browned. Stir in wine.

2. Combine onion mixture, broth, Worcestershire sauce, salt and thyme in **CROCK-POT®** slow cooker. Cover; cook on LOW 4 to 4½ hours.

3. Preheat broiler. Ladle soup into 4 oven-safe bowls; top with bread slice and cheese. Place beneath broiler until cheese melts and just starts to brown. Garnish with fresh thyme, if desired.

Makes 4 servings

Tip
To make broiling easier, place 4 empty oven-safe bowls on a rimmed baking sheet. Fill with soup and top with bread and cheese as directed above. The baking sheet makes it easier (and quicker, too) to slide the bowls of soup under the broiler.

New England Clam Chowder

6 slices bacon, diced
2 onions, chopped
5 cans (6½ ounces each) clams, drained and liquid reserved
6 medium red potatoes, cubed
2 tablespoons minced garlic
1 teaspoon black pepper
2 cans (12 ounces each) evaporated milk
  Salt, to taste
  Snipped fresh chives (optional)

1. Cook and stir bacon and onions in medium skillet until onions are tender. Place in **CROCK-POT®** slow cooker.

2. Add enough water to reserved clam liquid to make 3 cups. Pour into **CROCK-POT®** slow cooker, and add potatoes, garlic and pepper. Cover; cook on LOW 5 to 8 hours or HIGH 1 to 3 hours.

3. Turn **CROCK-POT®** slow cooker to LOW and mix in reserved clams and milk. Cover; cook 30 to 45 minutes. Adjust seasoning, if necessary, and garnish with snipped chives, if desired.

Makes 6 to 8 servings

Tip

*Shellfish and mollusks are delicate and should be added to the **CROCK-POT®** slow cooker during the last 15 to 30 minutes of the cooking time if you're using the HIGH heat setting, and during the last 30 to 45 minutes if you're using the LOW setting. This type of seafood overcooks easily, becoming tough and rubbery, so watch your cooking times, and cook only long enough for foods to be done.*

Simmering Hot and Sour Soup

2 cans (14½ ounces each) chicken broth
1 cup chopped cooked chicken or pork
4 ounces fresh shiitake mushroom caps, thinly sliced
½ cup thinly sliced bamboo shoots
3 tablespoons rice wine vinegar
2 tablespoons soy sauce
1½ teaspoons chili paste or 1 teaspoon hot chili oil
4 ounces firm tofu, well drained and cut into ½-inch pieces
2 teaspoons sesame oil
2 tablespoons cornstarch
2 tablespoons cold water
Chopped cilantro or sliced green onions

1. Combine broth, chicken, mushrooms, bamboo shoots, vinegar, soy sauce and chili paste in **CROCK-POT®** slow cooker. Cover; cook on LOW 3 to 4 hours or on HIGH 2 to 3 hours or until chicken is cooked through.

2. Stir in tofu and sesame oil. Combine cornstarch with water; mix well. Add to soup and mix in well. Cover; cook on HIGH 10 minutes or until soup has thickened. To serve, sprinkle with cilantro.

Makes 4 servings

Cannellini Minestrone Soup

- **4 cups chicken broth**
- **1 can (14½ ounces) diced tomatoes, undrained**
- **1 can (12 ounces) tomato-vegetable juice**
- **2 cups escarole, cut into ribbons**
- **1 cup chopped green onions**
- **1 cup chopped carrots**
- **1 cup chopped celery**
- **1 cup chopped potatoes**
- **¼ cup dried cannellini beans, sorted and rinsed**
- **2 tablespoons chopped fresh chives**
- **1 tablespoon chopped fresh flat-leaf parsley**
- **¼ teaspoon salt**
- **¼ teaspoon black pepper**
- **2 ounces uncooked ditalini pasta**

1. Place all ingredients except pasta in **CROCK-POT®** slow cooker. Stir well to combine. Cover; cook on LOW 6 to 8 hours or on HIGH 4 to 6 hours.

2. Add ditalini and stir again. Cover; cook 20 minutes before serving.

Makes 6 servings

Nana's Mini Meatball Soup

1 **pound ground beef**
1 **pound ground pork**
1½ **cups finely grated Pecorino Romano
or Parmesan cheese**
1 **cup Italian bread crumbs**
2 **eggs**
1 **bunch flat-leaf parsley
Kosher salt and black pepper**
3 **quarts chicken stock**
1 **bunch escarole, coarsely chopped**
½ **box (8 ounces) ditalini pasta, cooked**

1. Combine beef, pork, cheese, bread crumbs, eggs, parsley, salt and pepper in large bowl. Mix well by hand and roll into ¾-inch meatballs.

2. Add meatballs and chicken stock to **CROCK-POT®** slow cooker. Cook on LOW 9 hours or on HIGH 5 hours.

3. Add escarole and cook until escarole has wilted and is bright green and tender, about 15 minutes. Add cooked ditalini to soup and serve.

Makes 6 to 8 servings

Tip
Substitute spinach for escarole, if desired.

Greek Lemon and Rice Soup

- **3 cans (14 ounces each) chicken broth**
- **½ cup uncooked long-grain white rice (not converted or instant rice)**
- **3 egg yolks**
- **¼ cup fresh lemon juice**
- **¼ teaspoon salt**
- **⅛ teaspoon ground white pepper***
- **4 thin slices lemon (optional)**
- **4 teaspoons finely chopped parsley (optional)**

Substitute ground black pepper if desired.

1. Stir chicken broth and rice together in **CROCK-POT®** slow cooker. Cover and cook on HIGH 2 to 3 hours or until rice is cooked.

2. Turn to LOW. Whisk egg yolks and lemon juice together in medium bowl. Whisk large spoonful of hot rice mixture into egg yolk mixture. Whisk back into **CROCK-POT®** slow cooker.

3. Cook on LOW 10 minutes. Season with salt and pepper. Ladle soup into serving bowls and garnish each bowl with thin slice of lemon and 1 teaspoon chopped parsley, if desired.

Makes 4 servings

Note

Soup may be served hot or cold. To serve cold, allow soup to cool to room temperature. Cover and refrigerate up to 24 hours before serving.

Pizza Soup

2 cans (14½ ounces each) stewed tomatoes
  with Italian seasonings, undrained
2 cups beef broth
1 cup sliced mushrooms
1 small onion, chopped
1 tablespoon tomato paste
¼ teaspoon salt, or to taste
¼ teaspoon black pepper, or to taste
½ pound turkey Italian sausage, casings removed
  Shredded mozzarella cheese

1. Combine tomatoes with juice, broth, mushrooms, onion, tomato paste, salt and pepper in **CROCK-POT®** slow cooker.

2. Shape sausage into marble-size balls. Gently stir into soup mixture. Cover; cook on LOW 6 to 7 hours. Adjust salt and pepper, if necessary. Serve with cheese.

Makes 4 servings

Chicken Soup

6 cups chicken broth
1½ pounds boneless, skinless chicken breasts, cubed
2 cups sliced carrots
1 cup sliced mushrooms
1 red bell pepper, chopped
1 onion, chopped
2 tablespoons grated fresh ginger
3 teaspoons minced garlic
½ teaspoon crushed red pepper
Salt and black pepper, to taste

Place all ingredients in **CROCK-POT®** slow cooker. Cover; cook on LOW 6 to 7 hours or on HIGH 3 to 3½ hours.

Makes 4 to 6 servings

Wisconsin Beer and Cheese Soup

2 to 3 slices pumpernickel or rye bread
1 can (14½ ounces) chicken broth
1 cup beer
¼ cup finely chopped onion
2 cloves garlic, minced
¾ teaspoon dried thyme
6 ounces American cheese, shredded or diced
4 to 6 ounces sharp Cheddar cheese, shredded
1 cup milk
½ teaspoon paprika

1. Preheat oven to 425°F. Slice bread into ½-inch cubes; place on baking sheet. Bake 10 to 12 minutes, or until crisp, stirring once; set aside.

2. Combine broth, beer, onion, garlic and thyme in **CROCK-POT®** slow cooker. Cover; cook on LOW 4 hours.

3. Turn **CROCK-POT®** slow cooker to HIGH. Stir in cheeses, milk and paprika. Cover; cook 45 minutes to 1 hour, or until soup is hot and cheeses are melted. Stir soup well to blend cheeses. Ladle soup into bowls; top with croutons.

Makes 4 servings

Tip
Choose a light-tasting beer when making this soup. Hearty ales have a stronger flavor that might not please your family's taste buds.

Fresh Lime and Black Bean Soup

- **2 cans (15 ounces each) black beans, undrained**
- **1 can (14 ounces) reduced-sodium chicken broth**
- **1½ cups chopped onion**
- **1½ teaspoons chili powder**
- **¾ teaspoon ground cumin**
- **¼ teaspoon garlic powder**
- **⅛ to ¼ teaspoon red pepper flakes**
- **½ cup sour cream**
- **2 tablespoons extra-virgin olive oil**
- **2 tablespoons chopped cilantro**
- **1 medium lime, cut into wedges**

1. Coat **CROCK-POT®** slow cooker with nonstick cooking spray. Add beans, broth, onion, chili powder, cumin, garlic powder and pepper flakes. Cover; cook on LOW 7 hours or on HIGH 3½ hours, or until onion is very soft.

2. Process 1 cup soup mixture in blender until smooth and return to **CROCK-POT®** slow cooker. Stir, check consistency and repeat with additional 1 cup soup, as needed. Let stand 15 to 20 minutes before serving.

3. Ladle soup into 4 bowls. Divide sour cream, oil and cilantro evenly among servings. Squeeze juice from lime wedge over each.

Makes 4 servings

Tip

Brighten the flavor of dishes cooked in the *CROCK-POT®* slow cooker by adding fresh herbs or fresh lemon or lime juice before serving.

STEWS

Asian Beef Stew

     2   onions, cut into ¼-inch slices
    1½   pounds round steak, sliced thin across the grain
     2   stalks celery, sliced
     2   carrots, peeled and sliced or 1 cup peeled baby carrots
     1   cup sliced mushrooms
     1   cup orange juice
     1   cup beef broth
     ⅓   cup hoisin sauce
     2   tablespoons cornstarch
     1   to 2 teaspoons Chinese five-spice powder
         or curry powder
     1   cup frozen peas
         Hot cooked rice
         Chopped fresh cilantro (optional)

1. Place onions, beef, celery, carrots and mushrooms in **CROCK-POT®** slow cooker.

2. Combine orange juice, broth, hoisin sauce, cornstarch and five-spice powder in small bowl. Pour into **CROCK-POT®** slow cooker. Cover; cook on HIGH 5 hours or until beef is tender.

3. Stir in peas. Cook 20 minutes longer or until peas are tender. Serve with hot cooked rice, and garnish with cilantro, if desired.

Makes 6 servings

Jerk Pork and Sweet Potato Stew

    2 **tablespoons all-purpose flour**
    ¼ **teaspoon salt, or to taste**
    ¼ **teaspoon black pepper, or to taste**
    1¼ **pounds pork shoulder, cut into bite-size pieces**
    2 **tablespoons vegetable oil**
    1 **large sweet potato, peeled and diced**
    1 **cup frozen or canned corn**
    ¼ **cup minced green onions, green parts only, divided**
    1 **clove garlic, minced**
    ½ **medium Scotch bonnet chile or jalapeño pepper, cored, seeded and minced (about 1 teaspoon)***
    ⅛ **teaspoon ground allspice**
    1 **cup chicken broth**
    1 **tablespoon lime juice**
    2 **cups cooked rice (optional)**

*Scotch bonnet chiles and jalapeño peppers can sting and irritate the skin, so wear rubber gloves when handling and do not touch your eyes.

1. Combine flour, salt and pepper in resealable plastic food storage bag. Add pork and shake well to coat. Heat oil in large skillet over medium heat until hot. Add pork in a single layer (working in 2 batches, if necessary) and brown on both sides, about 5 minutes. Transfer to **CROCK-POT®** slow cooker.

2. Add sweet potato, corn, 2 tablespoons green onions, garlic, chile and allspice. Stir in broth. Cover; cook on LOW 5 to 6 hours.

3. Stir in lime juice and remaining 2 tablespoons green onions. Adjust salt and pepper to taste. Serve stew over cooked rice, if desired.

Makes 4 servings

Tip
To reduce the amount of fat in *CROCK-POT®* slow cooker meals, trim excess fat from meats and degrease canned broth before using.

Sweet and Sour Brisket Stew

    1 **jar (12 ounces) chili sauce**
1½ **to 2 tablespoons packed dark brown sugar**
1½ **tablespoons fresh lemon juice**
  ¼ **cup beef broth**
   1 **tablespoon Dijon mustard**
  ¼ **teaspoon paprika**
  ½ **teaspoon salt, or to taste**
  ¼ **teaspoon black pepper, or to taste**
   1 **clove garlic, minced**
   1 **small onion, chopped**
   1 **well-trimmed beef brisket, cut into 1-inch pieces***
   2 **large carrots, cut into ½-inch slices**
   1 **tablespoon all-purpose flour (optional)**

*Beef brisket has a thick layer of fat, which some supermarkets trim off. If the meat is well trimmed, buy 2½ pounds; if not, purchase 4 pounds, then trim and discard excess fat.

1. Combine chili sauce, 1½ tablespoons brown sugar, lemon juice, broth, mustard, paprika, salt and pepper in **CROCK-POT®** slow cooker. (Add remaining sugar, if desired, after tasting.)

2. Add garlic, onion, beef and carrots. Stir well to coat. Cover; cook on LOW 8 hours.

3. If thicker gravy is desired, combine 1 tablespoon flour and 3 tablespoons cooking liquid in small bowl. Add to **CROCK-POT®** slow cooker. Cover; cook on HIGH 10 minutes, or until thickened.

Makes 6 to 8 servings

New Mexican Green Chile Pork Stew

1½ pounds boneless pork shoulder, cut into 1-inch cubes
2 medium baking potatoes or sweet potatoes, peeled and cut into large chunks
1 cup chopped onion
1 can (4 ounces) diced green chiles
1 cup frozen corn
2 teaspoons sugar
2 teaspoons cumin or chili powder
1 teaspoon dried oregano
1 jar (16 ounces) salsa verde (green salsa)
   Hot cooked rice
¼ cup chopped fresh cilantro

1. Place pork, potatoes, onion, chiles and corn into **CROCK-POT®** slow cooker. Stir sugar, cumin and oregano into salsa and pour over pork and vegetables. Stir gently to mix.

2. Cover and cook on LOW 6 to 8 hours or on HIGH 4 to 5 hours, or until pork is tender. Serve stew over hot rice and garnish with cilantro.

Makes 6 servings

Tip

*Root vegetables such as potatoes can sometimes take longer to cook in a **CROCK-POT®** slow cooker than meat. Place uniformly cut vegetables on the bottom or along the sides of the **CROCK-POT®** slow cooker when possible.*

Traditional Cassoulet

1 small onion, finely chopped
2 cloves garlic, finely chopped
½ cup finely chopped peeled carrots
½ cup roughly chopped seeded tomatoes
1 can (about 15 ounces) cannellini beans, rinsed and drained
¼ cup bread crumbs
2 tablespoons finely chopped fresh marjoram leaves
2 tablespoons finely chopped fresh parsley leaves
2 tablespoons olive oil
1½ pounds chicken thighs
½ pound bulk pork sausage
½ cup dry white wine
½ cup chicken broth

1. Combine onion, garlic, carrots, tomatoes, beans, bread crumbs and fresh herbs in **CROCK-POT®** slow cooker. Set aside.

2. Heat olive oil in large skillet over medium-high heat. Add chicken (working in batches, if necessary) and cook 3 to 4 minutes per side or until brown. Place chicken on top of onion mixture. Add sausage to skillet. Cook, stirring to break up meat, until cooked through. Transfer sausage to **CROCK-POT®** slow cooker with slotted spoon.

3. Return skillet to medium-high heat. Add wine and chicken broth to skillet and stir to scrape up any browned bits. Bring to a boil and cook until liquid is reduced to about one third its original volume. Remove from heat.

4. Pour reduced liquid over contents of **CROCK-POT®** slow cooker. Cover and cook on LOW 6 to 7 hours or on HIGH 3½ hours.

Makes 4 servings

Greek Braised Beef Stew

¼ cup all-purpose flour

2 teaspoons Greek seasoning

¼ teaspoon salt, or to taste

¼ teaspoon black pepper, or to taste

2 pounds boneless beef stew meat or beef chuck roast, cut into 1-inch cubes

2 tablespoons olive oil

2 large onions, each cut into 8 wedges

1 container (10 ounces) grape or cherry tomatoes

1 jar (8 ounces) pitted kalamata olives, drained

8 sprigs fresh oregano, divided

1 lemon, divided

2 cups fat-free, reduced-sodium beef broth

1. Combine flour, Greek seasoning, salt and pepper in large resealable plastic food storage bag. Add beef, and shake to coat. Heat olive oil in large skillet over medium-high heat until hot. Add beef in single layer (working in 2 batches, if necessary) and brown on both sides, about 5 minutes. Transfer to **CROCK-POT®** slow cooker.

2. Add onions, tomatoes, olives, 4 sprigs oregano, juice of ½ lemon and broth. Cover; cook on HIGH 6 to 7 hours or until beef is tender. Add salt and pepper, if desired. Cut remaining ½ lemon into wedges and serve with stew. Garnish with remaining oregano.

Makes 6 servings

Tip

*Removing the lid from your **CROCK-POT®** slow cooker, even for just a few minutes to check on the progress of the dish inside, can allow significant amounts of heat to escape, requiring additional cooking time. Instead, try spinning or tapping the cover until the condensation falls off and allows you to see inside.*

Chipotle Chicken Stew

1 pound boneless, skinless chicken thighs, cut into cubes
1 can (15 ounces) navy beans, rinsed and drained
1 can (15 ounces) black beans, rinsed and drained
1 can (14½ ounces) crushed tomatoes, undrained
1½ cups chicken broth
½ cup orange juice
1 medium onion, diced
1 chipotle pepper in adobo sauce, minced
1 teaspoon salt
1 teaspoon ground cumin
1 bay leaf
Cilantro sprigs (optional)

1. Combine chicken, beans, tomatoes with juice, broth, orange juice, onion, chipotle pepper, salt, cumin and bay leaf in **CROCK-POT®** slow cooker.

2. Cover; cook on LOW 7 to 8 hours or on HIGH 3½ to 4 hours. Remove bay leaf before serving. Garnish with cilantro sprigs, if desired.

Makes 6 servings

Easy Beef Stew

- **2 pounds beef stew meat, cut into 1-inch cubes**
- **1 can (4 ounces) mushrooms**
- **1 envelope (1 ounce) dry onion soup mix**
- **⅓ cup red or white wine**
- **1 can (10 ounces) condensed cream of mushroom soup, undiluted**
- **Hot cooked noodles**

Combine all ingredients except noodles in **CROCK-POT®** slow cooker. Cover; cook on LOW 8 to 12 hours. Serve over noodles.

Makes 4 to 6 servings

Tip
*Browning the beef before cooking it in the **CROCK-POT®** slow cooker isn't necessary but helps to enhance the flavor and appearance of the stew. If you have the time, use nonstick cooking spray and brown the meat in a large skillet before placing it in the **CROCK-POT®** slow cooker; follow the recipe as written.*

Hearty Lentil Stew

1 cup dried lentils, rinsed and sorted
1 package (16 ounces) frozen green beans, thawed
2 cups cauliflower florets
1 cup chopped onion
1 cup baby carrots, cut into halves crosswise
3 cups fat-free reduced-sodium chicken broth
2 teaspoons ground cumin
¾ teaspoon ground ginger
1 can (15 ounces) chunky tomato sauce with garlic and herbs
½ cup dry-roasted peanuts

1. Place lentils in **CROCK-POT®** slow cooker. Top with green beans, cauliflower, onion and carrots.

2. Combine broth, cumin and ginger in large bowl; mix well. Pour over vegetables in **CROCK-POT®** slow cooker. Cover; cook on LOW 9 to 11 hours.

3. Stir in tomato sauce. Cover; cook on LOW 10 minutes. Ladle stew into bowls. Sprinkle peanuts evenly over each serving.

Makes 6 servings

Chicken and Sweet Potato Stew

- **4 boneless, skinless chicken breasts, cut into bite-size pieces**
- **2 medium sweet potatoes, peeled and cubed**
- **2 medium Yukon Gold potatoes, peeled and cubed**
- **2 medium carrots, peeled and cut into ½-inch slices**
- **1 can (28 ounces) whole stewed tomatoes**
- **1 teaspoon salt**
- **1 teaspoon paprika**
- **1 teaspoon celery seeds**
- **½ teaspoon freshly ground black pepper**
- **⅛ teaspoon ground cinnamon**
- **⅛ teaspoon ground nutmeg**
- **1 cup nonfat, low-sodium chicken broth**
- **¼ cup fresh basil, chopped**

Combine all ingredients except basil in **CROCK-POT®** slow cooker. Cover; cook on LOW 6 to 8 hours or on HIGH 3 to 4 hours. Sprinkle with basil just before serving.

Makes 6 servings

Chicken Stew

- **4 to 5 cups chopped cooked chicken**
- **1 can (28 ounces) whole tomatoes, cut up, undrained**
- **2 large red potatoes, cut into 1-inch pieces**
- **8 ounces fresh okra, sliced**
- **1 large onion, chopped**
- **1 can (14 ounces) cream-style corn**
- **½ cup ketchup**
- **½ cup barbecue sauce**

Combine chicken, tomatoes with juice, potatoes, okra and onion in **CROCK-POT®** slow cooker. Cover; cook on LOW 6 to 8 hours or until potatoes are tender. Add corn, ketchup and barbecue sauce. Cover; cook on HIGH 30 minutes.

Makes 6 servings

Beef Stew with Molasses and Raisins

- ⅓ **cup all-purpose flour**
- 2 **teaspoons salt, divided**
- 1½ **teaspoons black pepper, divided**
- 2 **pounds beef for stew, cut into 1½-inch pieces**
- 5 **tablespoons oil, divided**
- 2 **medium onions, sliced**
- 1 **can (28 ounces) diced tomatoes, drained**
- 1 **cup beef broth**
- 3 **tablespoons molasses**
- 2 **tablespoons cider vinegar**
- 4 **cloves garlic, minced**
- 2 **teaspoons dried thyme**
- 1 **teaspoon celery salt**
- 1 **bay leaf**
- 8 **ounces baby carrots, cut in half lengthwise**
- 2 **parsnips, diced**
- ½ **cup golden raisins**

1. Combine flour, 1½ teaspoons salt and 1 teaspoon pepper in large bowl. Toss meat in flour mixture. Heat 2 tablespoons oil in large skillet or Dutch oven over medium-high heat until hot. Add half of beef and brown on all sides. Set aside browned beef and repeat with 2 additional tablespoons oil and remaining beef.

2. Add remaining 1 tablespoon oil to skillet. Add onions and cook, stirring to loosen any browned bits, about 5 minutes. Add tomatoes, broth, molasses, vinegar, garlic, thyme, celery salt, bay leaf and remaining ½ teaspoon salt and ½ teaspoon pepper. Bring to a boil. Add browned beef and boil 1 minute.

3. Transfer mixture to **CROCK-POT®** slow cooker. Cover; cook on LOW 5 hours or on HIGH 2½ hours. Add carrots, parsnips and raisins. Cook 1 to 2 hours longer or until vegetables are tender. Remove and discard bay leaf.

Makes 6 to 8 servings

Quatro Frijoles con Pollo Cantaro

- 1 **cup pitted black olives, drained**
- 1 **pound boneless, skinless chicken breast, cubed***
- 1 **can (16 ounces) garbanzo beans, rinsed and drained**
- 1 **can (16 ounces) Great Northern or navy beans, rinsed and drained**
- 1 **can (15 ounces) cannellini beans, rinsed and drained**
- 1 **can (16 ounces) red kidney beans, rinsed and drained**
- 1 **can (7 ounces) chopped mild green chilies, drained**
- 2 **cups chicken stock, plus extra as needed**
- 2 **tablespoons canola or olive oil**
- 1 **cup minced onion**
- 2 **teaspoons minced garlic**
- 1½ **teaspoons ground cumin**
   Hot sauce, to taste
   Salt and black pepper, to taste
- 2 **cups crushed corn chips**
- 6 **ounces Monterey Jack cheese, grated**

Substitute turkey, pork or beef for the chicken, as desired.

1. Combine olives, chicken, beans, chilies and chicken stock in **CROCK-POT®** slow cooker. Mix well; set aside.

2. Heat oil in large skillet over medium-high heat. Cook onion, garlic and cumin until onion is soft, stirring frequently. Add to chicken mixture. Cover; cook on LOW 4 to 5 hours. Check liquid about halfway through, adding more hot broth as needed.

3. Taste and add hot sauce, salt and pepper. Serve in warm bowls and garnish with corn chips and cheese.

Makes 6 servings

Cod Fish Stew

½ **pound bacon, coarsely chopped**
1 **large carrot, diced**
1 **large onion, diced**
2 **stalks celery, diced**
2 **cloves garlic, minced**
   Kosher salt and black pepper
1 **can (28 ounces) plum tomatoes, drained**
3 **tablespoons tomato paste**
½ **cup white wine**
3 **tablespoons chopped flat-leaf parsley**
3 **cups water**
2 **cups clam juice or fish stock**
3 **saffron threads**
2 **potatoes, peeled and diced**
2½ **pounds fresh cod, skinned and cut into bite-size pieces**

1. In skillet over medium-high heat, cook bacon until crisp. Remove with slotted spoon. Add carrot, onion, celery and garlic to skillet, season with salt and pepper and cook, stirring, until vegetables soften.

2. Place bacon and vegetables in **CROCK-POT®** slow cooker. Stir in tomatoes, tomato paste, wine, parsley, water, clam juice, saffron and potatoes. Cook on LOW 6 to 7 hours or on HIGH 3 to 4 hours, or until potatoes are tender.

3. Add cod and cook 10 to 20 minutes, or until cod is just cooked through.

Makes 6 to 8 servings

Note

Cod is a great fish to use for a soup or stew. The thick creamy white fish becomes a hearty meal when paired with bacon and tomato.

DESSERTS & BEVERAGES

Slow Cooking Desserts & Beverages

Baked goods in a slow cooker

If you wish to prepare bread, cakes, or pudding cakes in a slow cooker, you may want to purchase a covered, vented metal cake pan accessory for your slow cooker. You can also use any straight-sided soufflé dish or deep cake pan that will fit into the ceramic insert of your unit. Baked goods can be prepared directly in the insert; they can be a little difficult to remove from the insert, so follow the recipe directions carefully. *(See Foil Handles below for tips on removing soufflé dishes and cake pans from your slow cooker.)*

High altitude adjustments

If you live at an altitude above 3,500 feet, you will need to make some adjustments. First, contact the United States Department of Agriculture Extensive Service in your state for advice on high-altitude cooking. If they don't have specific information about slow cooking at high altitudes, you will have to do some experimenting. Everything will take longer to cook, so plan for that. Tough meats take longer to tenderize at high altitudes, sometimes much longer; try cooking on the HIGH heat setting instead of LOW. Root vegetables take longer to cook as

well; cut them into smaller pieces than the recipe suggests for quicker cooking.

Beverages

Your **CROCK-POT®** slow cooker can make serving wonderful warming beverages simpler than ever. You can easily make enough hot cocoa or mulled cider to satisfy a crowd. What's more, your slow cooker can be set to keep any bracing beverage at exactly the right temperature.

Foil Handles

Some recipes call for using foil handles to lift a dish or a meatloaf out of the slow cooker. Foil handles are easy to make; just follow these easy instructions:

Tear off three 18 × 3-inch strips of heavy-duty foil. Crisscross the strips so they resemble the spokes of a wheel. Place the dish or food in the center of the strips. Pull foil strips up and over, and place into the slow cooker. Leave them in while you cook so you can easily lift the item out again when it is ready.

DESSERTS

Bananas Foster

12 **bananas, cut into quarters**
 1 **cup flaked coconut**
 1 **teaspoon ground cinnamon**
½ **teaspoon salt**
 1 **cup dark corn syrup**
⅔ **cup butter, melted**
 2 **teaspoons grated lemon peel**
¼ **cup lemon juice**
 2 **teaspoons rum**
12 **slices pound cake**
 1 **quart vanilla ice cream**

Combine bananas and coconut in **CROCK-POT®** slow cooker. Combine cinnamon, salt, corn syrup, butter, lemon peel, lemon juice and rum in medium bowl; pour over bananas. Cover; cook on LOW 1 to 2 hours. To serve, arrange bananas on pound cake slices. Top with ice cream and pour on warm sauce.

Makes 12 servings

Strawberry Rhubarb Crisp

FRUIT
- **4 cups sliced hulled strawberries**
- **4 cups diced rhubarb (about 5 stalks), cut into ½-inch dice**
- **1½ cups granulated sugar**
- **2 tablespoons lemon juice**
- **1½ tablespoons cornstarch, plus water (optional)**

TOPPING
- **1 cup all-purpose flour**
- **1 cup old-fashioned oats**
- **½ cup granulated sugar**
- **½ cup packed brown sugar**
- **½ teaspoon ground ginger**
- **½ teaspoon ground nutmeg**
- **½ cup butter (1 stick), cut into pieces**
- **½ cup sliced almonds, toasted***

*To toast almonds, spread in single layer on baking sheet. Bake in preheated 350°F oven 8 to 10 minutes or until golden brown, stirring frequently.

1. Coat **CROCK-POT®** slow cooker with nonstick cooking spray. Place strawberries, rhubarb, granulated sugar and lemon juice in **CROCK-POT®** slow cooker and mix well. Cook on HIGH 1½ hours or until fruit is tender.

2. If fruit is dry after cooking, add a little water. If fruit has too much liquid, mix cornstarch with a little water and stir into **CROCK-POT®** slow cooker. Cover and cook on HIGH an additional 15 minutes or until cooking liquid is thickened.

3. Preheat oven to 375°F. Prepare topping: Combine flour, oats, sugars, ginger and nutmeg in medium bowl. Cut in butter using pastry cutter or 2 knives until mixture resembles coarse crumbs. Stir in almonds.

4. Remove lid from **CROCK-POT®** slow cooker and gently sprinkle topping onto fruit. Transfer stoneware to oven. Bake 15 to 20 minutes or until topping begins to brown.

Makes 8 servings

Rum and Cherry Cola Fudge Spoon Cake

CAKE

- ½ cup cola
- ½ cup dried sour cherries
- 1 cup chocolate milk
- ½ cup (1 stick) unsalted butter, melted
- 2 teaspoons vanilla
- 1½ cups all-purpose flour
- ½ cup ground sweet chocolate
- ½ cup granulated sugar
- 2½ teaspoons baking powder
- ½ teaspoon salt

TOPPING

- 1¼ cups vanilla cola
- ¼ cup dark rum
- ½ cup ground sweet chocolate
- ½ cup granulated sugar
- ½ cup packed brown sugar

1. Coat **CROCK-POT®** slow cooker with nonstick cooking spray. Bring cola and dried cherries to a boil in saucepan. Remove from heat; let stand 30 minutes.

2. Combine chocolate milk, melted butter and vanilla in small bowl. Combine flour, ground chocolate, granulated sugar, baking powder and salt in medium bowl; stir to mix well. Make a well in center of dry ingredients; add milk mixture and stir until smooth. Stir cherry mixture into batter. Pour into **CROCK-POT®** slow cooker.

3. Prepare topping: Bring vanilla cola and rum to a boil in saucepan. Remove from heat. Add ground chocolate and sugars; stir until smooth. Gently pour over batter. Do not stir. Cover; cook on HIGH 2½ hours or until cake is puffed and top layer has set.

4. Turn off **CROCK-POT®** slow cooker. Let stand, covered, 30 minutes. Serve warm. Garnish as desired.

Makes 8 to 10 servings

Plum Bread Pudding

1 loaf (1 pound) sliced egg bread, lightly toasted*

2 tablespoons unsalted butter, divided

12 large unpeeled Italian plums, pitted and cut into wedges (about 4 cups total)

1½ cups plus 2 tablespoons sugar, divided

3 cups half-and-half

10 eggs

1¼ cups milk

2 teaspoons vanilla

¾ teaspoon salt

¾ teaspoon ground cinnamon

Sweetened whipped cream or vanilla ice cream (optional)

Use an egg-rich bread, such as challah, for best results. For a more delicate bread pudding, substitute cinnamon rolls or plain Danish rolls.

1. Lightly coat inside of 6-quart **CROCK-POT**® slow cooker with cooking spray.

2. Cut toasted bread into 1-inch pieces; set aside.

3. Melt 1 tablespoon butter in large skillet over medium-high heat. Add half sliced plums. Sprinkle with 1 tablespoon sugar. Cook 2 minutes or until plums are pulpy and give off juices. Pour plums and juices into medium bowl; repeat with remaining 1 tablespoon butter, remaining plums and 1 tablespoon sugar. Set aside to cool slightly.

4. Beat together half-and-half, eggs, milk, remaining 1½ cups sugar, vanilla, salt and cinnamon in large bowl. Stir in bread cubes, plums and any accumulated juices. Spoon into prepared **CROCK-POT**® slow cooker. Cover and cook on HIGH 3 hours or until pudding is firm when gently shaken and thin knife inserted halfway between center and edge comes out clean. Remove insert from base and cool 15 minutes. Serve with whipped cream or ice cream, if desired.

Makes 12 to 16 servings

Peach Bread Pudding

If fresh plums are not available, substitute 9 large peaches, peeled, pitted and cut into wedges or 4 cups frozen sliced peaches, thawed (juices reserved).

Homestyle Apple Brown Betty

- 6 **cups of your favorite cooking apples, peeled, cored and cut into eighths**
- 1 **cup bread crumbs**
- 1 **teaspoon ground cinnamon**
- 1 **teaspoon ground nutmeg**
- ⅛ **teaspoon salt**
- ¾ **cup packed brown sugar**
- ½ **cup (1 stick) butter or margarine, melted**
- ¼ **cup finely chopped walnuts**

1. Lightly grease **CROCK-POT®** slow cooker. Place apples on bottom.

2. Combine bread crumbs, cinnamon, nutmeg, salt, brown sugar, butter and walnuts, and spread over apples.

3. Cover; cook on LOW 3 to 4 hours or on HIGH 2 hours.

Makes 8 servings

Tip
Expecting a crowd? Just double the amount of all the ingredients and prepare in a 5-, 6- or 7-quart CROCK-POT® slow cooker.

Classic Baked Apples

- ¼ **cup packed dark brown sugar**
- 2 **tablespoons golden raisins**
- 1 **teaspoon grated lemon peel**
- 6 **small to medium baking apples, washed and cored**
- 1 **teaspoon ground cinnamon**
- 2 **tablespoons butter, cut into small pieces**
- ¼ **cup orange juice**
- ¼ **cup water**
  Whipped cream (optional)

1. Combine brown sugar, raisins and lemon peel in small bowl. Fill core of each apple with mixture. Place apples in **CROCK-POT®** slow cooker. Sprinkle with cinnamon and dot with butter. Pour orange juice and water over apples. Cover; cook on LOW 7 to 9 hours or on HIGH 2½ to 3½ hours.

2. To serve, place apples in individual bowls. Top with sauce. Garnish with whipped cream, if desired.

Makes 6 servings

Cherry Rice Pudding

- **1½ cups milk**
- **1 cup hot cooked rice**
- **3 eggs, beaten**
- **½ cup sugar**
- **¼ cup dried cherries or cranberries**
- **½ teaspoon almond extract**
- **¼ teaspoon salt**
- **Ground nutmeg, for garnish**

1. Combine all ingredients in large bowl. Pour into greased 1½-quart casserole dish. Cover dish with buttered aluminum foil, butter side down.

2. Place rack in **CROCK-POT®** slow cooker and pour in 1 cup water. Place casserole on rack. Cover; cook on LOW 4 to 5 hours.

3. Remove casserole from **CROCK-POT®** slow cooker. Let stand 15 minutes before serving. Garnish with nutmeg, if desired.

Makes 6 servings

Cinnamon-Ginger Poached Pears

3 cups water
1 cup sugar
10 slices fresh ginger
2 whole cinnamon sticks
1 tablespoon chopped candied ginger (optional)
6 Bosc or Anjou pears, peeled and cored

1. Combine water, sugar, ginger, cinnamon and candied ginger, if desired, in **CROCK-POT®** slow cooker. Add pears. Cover; cook on LOW 4 to 6 hours or on HIGH 1½ to 2 hours.

2. Remove pears. Cook syrup, uncovered, 30 minutes or until thickened.

Makes 6 servings

Easy Peach Buckle

- 2 **packages (16 ounces each) frozen peach slices, thawed or 5 cups fresh peach slices**
- ¼ **cup granulated sugar**
- 1¾ **cups plus all-purpose flour**
- ½ **cup packed brown sugar**
- 2 **teaspoons baking powder**
- 1 **teaspoon ground cinnamon**
- 1 **teaspoon baking soda**
- ¼ **teaspoon salt**
- 1⅓ **cups buttermilk**
- 6 **tablespoons canola oil**
- 1 **teaspoon vanilla**

1. Lightly coat inside of 4½-quart **CROCK-POT**® slow cooker with cooking spray.

2. Toss peaches with granulated sugar; set aside.

3. Combine flour, brown sugar, baking powder, cinnamon, baking soda and salt in medium bowl. Combine buttermilk, oil and vanilla in small bowl; mix well. Stir into flour mixture just until blended.

4. Spread batter evenly in prepared **CROCK-POT**® slow cooker. Arrange peaches on batter. Cover and cook on HIGH 2½ hours or until buckle springs back when touched. Serve warm.

Makes 12 servings

Mixed Berry Cobbler

  1 **package (16 ounces) frozen mixed berries**
 ¾ **cup granulated sugar**
  2 **tablespoons quick-cooking tapioca**
  2 **teaspoons grated lemon peel**
1½ **cups all-purpose flour**
 ½ **cup packed light brown sugar**
2¼ **teaspoons baking powder**
 ¼ **teaspoon ground nutmeg**
 ¾ **cup milk**
 ⅓ **cup butter, melted**
    Vanilla ice cream or whipped cream (optional)

1. Coat **CROCK-POT®** slow cooker with nonstick cooking spray. Stir together berries, granulated sugar, tapioca and lemon peel in medium bowl. Transfer to **CROCK-POT®** slow cooker.

2. For topping, combine flour, brown sugar, baking powder and nutmeg in medium bowl. Add milk and butter; stir just until blended. Drop spoonfuls of dough on top of berry mixture. Cover; cook on LOW 4 hours. Uncover; let stand about 30 minutes. Serve with ice cream, if desired.

Makes 8 servings

Tip

Cobblers are easy year-round favorites. Experiment with whatever fruit is in season. We recommend combinations of pears, plums, peaches, rhubarb or your favorite berries.

Rustic Peach-Oat Crumble

- 8 **cups frozen sliced peaches, thawed and juice reserved**
- ¾ **cup packed brown sugar, divided**
- 1½ **tablespoons cornstarch**
- 1 **tablespoon lemon juice (optional)**
- 1½ **teaspoons vanilla**
- ½ **teaspoon almond extract**
- 1 **cup quick oats**
- ¼ **cup all-purpose flour**
- ¼ **cup granulated sugar**
- 1 **teaspoon ground cinnamon**
- ¼ **teaspoon salt**
- ½ **cup (1 stick) cold butter, cut into small pieces**

1. Lightly coat inside of 4½-quart **CROCK-POT®** slow cooker with cooking spray.

2. Combine peaches with juice, ½ cup brown sugar, cornstarch, lemon juice, if desired, vanilla and almond extract in medium bowl. Toss until peaches are well-coated. Transfer to prepared **CROCK-POT®** slow cooker.

3. Combine oats, flour, remaining ¼ cup brown sugar, granulated sugar, cinnamon and salt in medium bowl. Cut in butter with pastry blender or 2 knives until mixture resembles coarse crumbs. Sprinkle over peaches. Cover and cook on HIGH 1½ hours or until bubbly at edge. Remove insert from base and cool 20 minutes.

Makes about 8 servings

Italian Cheesecake

  6 **graham crackers, crushed to fine crumbs**
  2 **tablespoons packed brown sugar**
  2 **tablespoons unsalted butter, melted**
  2 **packages (8 ounces each) cream cheese**
1½ **cups granulated sugar**
  1 **container (15 ounces) ricotta cheese**
  2 **cups sour cream**
  1 **teaspoon vanilla**
  4 **eggs**
  3 **tablespoons cornstarch**
  3 **tablespoons all-purpose flour**
     Fresh strawberries (optional)
     Fresh mint (optional)

1. Line round 4½-quart **CROCK-POT®** slow cooker with with foil (see note below).
2. Combine graham crackers and brown sugar in bowl. Stir in melted butter until crumbs hold shape when pinched. Pat firmly into prepared **CROCK-POT®** slow cooker. Refrigerate until needed.
3. Beat cream cheese and granulated sugar in large bowl with electric mixer at medium speed until smooth. Add ricotta, sour cream and vanilla; beat until blended. Add eggs 1 at a time beating after each addition until well blended. Beat in cornstarch and flour. Pour filling into prepared crust. Cover and cook on LOW 3 to 4 hours or until cheesecake is nearly set.
4. Turn off **CROCK-POT®** slow cooker; remove lid, cover top of stoneware with clean kitchen towel and replace lid. Cool for 1 hour, then remove stoneware from base; cool completely in covered stoneware. Tranfer whole cheesecake to serving plate using foil as handle. Cover; refrigerate until serving. Serve garnished with strawberries and mint, if desired.

Makes 16 servings

Note

Lining the interior with foil allows you to remove the entire cheesecake and cut it into traditional wedges for serving. To line CROCK-POT® slow cooker with foil, remove the stoneware from the base and place upside-down on work surface. Tear off a 24-inch long piece of 18-inch-wide, heavy-duty foil. Place shiny-side down on top of upside-down stoneware. Smooth foil to stoneware, folding and tucking as necessary to fit. Remove foil, turn stoneware right-side up and place foil inside it. Smooth foil as much as possible to interior of stoneware, then lightly coat with nonstick cooking spray.

BEVERAGES

Warm and Spicy Fruit Punch

4	cinnamon sticks
1	orange, washed
1	square (8 inches) double-thickness cheesecloth
1	teaspoon whole allspice
½	teaspoon whole cloves
7	cups water
1	can (12 ounces) frozen cran-raspberry juice concentrate, thawed
1	can (6 ounces) frozen lemonade concentrate, thawed
2	cans (5½ ounces each) apricot nectar

1. Break cinnamon into pieces. Using vegetable peeler, remove strips of orange peel. Squeeze juice from orange; set juice aside.

2. Rinse cheesecloth; squeeze out water. Wrap cinnamon, orange peel, allspice and cloves in cheesecloth. Tie bag securely with cotton string or strip of cheesecloth.

3. Combine reserved orange juice, water, concentrates and apricot nectar in **CROCK-POT**® slow cooker; add spice bag. Cover; cook on LOW 5 to 6 hours. Remove and discard spice bag before serving.

Makes about 14 servings

Tip

To keep punch warm during a party, place your CROCK-POT® slow cooker on the buffet table, and set it to LOW or WARM.

Viennese Coffee

3 cups strong freshly brewed hot coffee
3 tablespoons chocolate syrup
1 teaspoon sugar
⅓ cup whipping cream
¼ cup crème de cacao or Irish cream (optional)
Whipped cream (optional)
Chocolate shavings (optional)

1. Combine coffee, chocolate syrup and sugar in **CROCK-POT®** slow cooker. Cover and cook on LOW 2 to 2½ hours. Stir in whipping cream and crème de cacao, if desired. Cover and cook 30 minutes or until heated through.

2. Ladle coffee into coffee cups. Top with whipped cream and chocolate shavings.

Makes 4 servings

Spiced Apple Tea

3 bags cinnamon herbal tea
3 cups boiling water
2 cups unsweetened apple juice
6 whole cloves
1 cinnamon stick

Place tea bags in **CROCK-POT®** slow cooker. Pour boiling water over tea bags; cover and let stand 10 minutes. Remove and discard tea bags. Add apple juice, cloves and cinnamon stick to **CROCK-POT®** slow cooker. Cover; cook on LOW 2 to 3 hours. Remove and discard cloves and cinnamon stick. Serve warm in mugs.

Makes 4 servings

Viennese Coffee

Cinnamon Latté

6 cups double-strength brewed coffee*
2 cups half-and-half
1 cup sugar
1 teaspoon vanilla
3 cinnamon sticks, plus additional for garnish
   Whipped cream (optional)

*Double the amount of coffee grounds normally used to brew coffee. Or, substitute 8 teaspoons instant coffee dissolved in 6 cups boiling water.

1. Blend coffee, half-and-half, sugar and vanilla in 3- to 4-quart **CROCK-POT**® slow cooker. Add cinnamon sticks. Cover; cook on HIGH 3 hours.

2. Remove cinnamon sticks. Serve latté in tall coffee mugs with dollop of whipped cream and cinnamon stick, if desired.

Makes 6 to 8 servings

Hot Mulled Cider

½ **gallon apple cider**
½ **cup packed light brown sugar**
1½ **teaspoons balsamic or cider vinegar (optional)**
1 **teaspoon vanilla**
1 **cinnamon stick**
6 **whole cloves**
½ **cup applejack or bourbon (optional)**

Combine all ingredients except applejack in **CROCK-POT®** slow cooker. Cover; cook on LOW 5 to 6 hours. Remove and discard cinnamon stick and cloves. Stir in applejack just before serving, if desired. Serve hot in mugs.

Makes 16 servings

Hot Tropics Sipper

4	cups pineapple juice
2	cups apple juice
1	container (about 11 ounces) apricot nectar
3	whole cinnamon sticks
6	whole cloves
½	cup packed dark brown sugar
1	medium lemon, thinly sliced
1	medium orange, thinly sliced
	Additional lemon or orange slices, for garnish

Place all ingredients except garnish in **CROCK-POT®** slow cooker. Cover; cook on HIGH 3½ to 4 hours, or until very fragrant. Strain immediately (beverage will turn bitter if fruit and spices remain after cooking is complete). Serve with fresh slices of lemon or orange, if desired.

Makes 8 servings

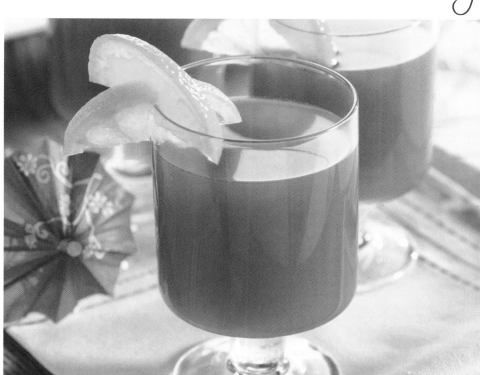

Chai Tea

2	quarts (8 cups) water
8	bags black tea
¾	cup sugar*
16	whole cloves
16	whole cardamom seeds, pods removed (optional)
5	cinnamon sticks
8	slices fresh ginger
1	cup milk

Chai tea is typically sweet. For less-sweet tea, reduce sugar to ½ cup.

1. Combine water, tea, sugar, cloves, cardamom, if desired, cinnamon and ginger in **CROCK-POT®** slow cooker. Cover; cook on HIGH 2 to 2½ hours.

2. Strain mixture; discard solids. (At this point, tea may be covered and refrigerated up to 3 days.)

3. Stir in milk just before serving. Serve warm or chilled.

Makes 8 to 10 servings

Mulled Cranberry Tea

- **2 tea bags**
- **1 cup boiling water**
- **1 bottle (48 ounces) cranberry juice**
- **½ cup dried cranberries (optional)**
- **⅓ cup sugar**
- **1 large lemon, cut into ¼-inch slices**
- **4 cinnamon sticks**
- **6 whole cloves**
  Additional cinnamon sticks or thin lemon slices (optional)

1. Place tea bags in **CROCK-POT®** slow cooker. Pour boiling water over tea bags; cover and let steep 5 minutes. Remove and discard tea bags.

2. Stir in cranberry juice, cranberries, if desired, sugar, lemon slices, 4 cinnamon sticks and cloves. Cover; cook on LOW 2 to 3 hours or on HIGH 1 to 2 hours.

3. Remove and discard cooked lemon slices, cinnamon sticks and cloves. Serve in warm mug with cinnamon stick or fresh lemon slice, if desired.

Makes 8 servings

Tip

*The flavor and aroma of crushed or ground herbs and spices may lessen during a longer cooking time. So, for slow cooking in your **CROCK-POT®** slow cooker, you may use whole herbs and spices. Be sure to taste and adjust seasoning with additional sugar or lemon juice before serving, if necessary.*

Mucho Mocha Cocoa

- **1 cup chocolate syrup**
- **⅓ cup instant coffee granules**
- **2 tablespoons sugar (or more to taste)**
- **2 whole cinnamon sticks**
- **1 quart whole milk**
- **1 quart half-and-half**

Combine all ingredients in **CROCK-POT®** slow cooker. Stir until well blended. Cover and cook on LOW 3 hours. Serve hot in mugs.

Makes 9 servings

Tip

This is great for a party. If desired, add 1 ounce of rum or whisky to each serving.

Spiced Citrus Tea

4 **tea bags**
Peel of 1 orange
4 **cups boiling water**
3 **tablespoons honey**
2 **cans (6 ounces each) orange-pineapple juice**
3 **star anise**
3 **cinnamon sticks**
Strawberries, raspberries or kiwis (optional)

Place tea bags, orange peel and boiling water in **CROCK-POT®** slow cooker; cover and let steep 10 minutes. Remove and discard tea bags and orange peel. Add remaining ingredients. Cover; cook on LOW 3 hours. Garnish as desired.

Makes 6 servings

Triple Delicious Hot Chocolate

⅓ cup sugar

¼ cup unsweetened cocoa powder

¼ teaspoon salt

3 cups milk, divided

¾ teaspoon vanilla

1 cup heavy cream

1 square (1 ounce) bittersweet chocolate

1 square (1 ounce) white chocolate

¾ cup whipped cream

6 teaspoons mini chocolate chips
or shaved bittersweet chocolate

1. Combine sugar, cocoa, salt and ½ cup milk in medium bowl. Beat until smooth. Transfer to **CROCK-POT®** slow cooker. Add remaining 2½ cups milk and vanilla; stir in. Cover; cook on LOW 2 hours.

2. Add cream. Cover; cook on LOW 10 minutes. Stir in bittersweet and white chocolates until melted.

3. Pour hot chocolate into 6 coffee cups. Top each serving with 2 tablespoons whipped cream and 1 teaspoon chocolate chips.

Makes 6 servings

INDEX

INDEX

C

Mucho Mocha Cocoa, p. 181

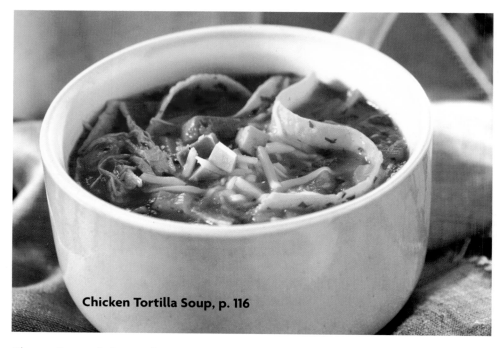

Chicken Tortilla Soup, p. 116

INDEX

Homestyle Apple Brown Betty, p. 164

INDEX

Mango Ginger Pork Roast, p. 66

INDEX

Classic Spaghetti, p. 16

INDEX

Greek-Style Chicken, p. 51

INDEX

METRIC CHART

VOLUME MEASUREMENTS (dry)

$1/8$ teaspoon = 0.5 mL
$1/4$ teaspoon = 1 mL
$1/2$ teaspoon = 2 mL
$3/4$ teaspoon = 4 mL
1 teaspoon = 5 mL
1 tablespoon = 15 mL
2 tablespoons = 30 mL
$1/4$ cup = 60 mL
$1/3$ cup = 75 mL
$1/2$ cup = 125 mL
$2/3$ cup = 150 mL
$3/4$ cup = 175 mL
1 cup = 250 mL
2 cups = 1 pint = 500 mL
3 cups = 750 mL
4 cups = 1 quart = 1 L

VOLUME MEASUREMENTS (fluid)

1 fluid ounce (2 tablespoons) = 30 mL
4 fluid ounces ($1/2$ cup) = 125 mL
8 fluid ounces (1 cup) = 250 mL
12 fluid ounces ($1 1/2$ cups) = 375 mL
16 fluid ounces (2 cups) = 500 mL

WEIGHTS (mass)

$1/2$ ounce = 15 g
1 ounce = 30 g
3 ounces = 90 g
4 ounces = 120 g
8 ounces = 225 g
10 ounces = 285 g
12 ounces = 360 g
16 ounces = 1 pound = 450 g

DIMENSIONS

$1/16$ inch = 2 mm
$1/8$ inch = 3 mm
$1/4$ inch = 6 mm
$1/2$ inch = 1.5 cm
$3/4$ inch = 2 cm
1 inch = 2.5 cm

OVEN TEMPERATURES

250°F = 120°C
275°F = 140°C
300°F = 150°C
325°F = 160°C
350°F = 180°C
375°F = 190°C
400°F = 200°C
425°F = 220°C
450°F = 230°C

BAKING PAN AND DISH EQUIVALENTS

Utensil	Size in Inches	Size in Centimeters	Volume	Metric Volume
Baking or Cake Pan (square or rectangular)	8×8×2	20×20×5	8 cups	2 L
	9×9×2	23×23×5	10 cups	2.5 L
	13×9×2	33×23×5	12 cups	3 L
Loaf Pan	8½×4½×2½	21×11×6	6 cups	1.5 L
	9×9×3	23×13×7	8 cups	2 L
Round Layer Cake Pan	8×1½	20×4	4 cups	1 L
	9×1½	23×4	5 cups	1.25 L
Pie Plate	8×1½	20×4	4 cups	1 L
	9×1½	23×4	5 cups	1.25 L
Baking Dish or Casserole			1 quart/4 cups	1 L
			1½ quart/6 cups	1.5 L
			2 quart/8 cups	2 L
			3 quart/12 cups	3 L